Hello, Down There

A Guide to Healing Chronic Pelvic and Sexual Pain

Alexandra T. Milspaw, PhD, MEd

This book is intended as a reference volume only, not as a medical manual. The information given here is designed to inspire and inform. It is not intended as a substitute for any treatment that may have been prescribed by your doctor. If you suspect that you have a medical problem, we urge you to seek competent medical help.

Internet addresses given in this book were accurate at the time it went to press.

Printed in the United States of America
Published in Hellertown, PA

Cover and interior design by Anna Magruder
Illustrations by Samuel V. Couchara
Library of Congress Control Number 2022914616
ISBN: 978-1-958711-10-1
2 4 6 8 10 9 7 5 3 1

For more information or to place bulk orders, contact the publisher at Jennifer@BrightCommunications.net.

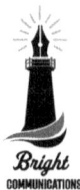

Bright
COMMUNICATIONS

BrightCommunications.net

This book is dedicated to my clients, who continue to inspire my work through their resilience and demonstration of the powerful human body, mind, heart, and spirit to overcome some of the most abhorrent traumas and consequential pain I have witnessed. You continue to fuel my passion and inspire my belief in our ability to return to our natural state of well-being.

Contents

Acknowledgments

I wish to express my deep gratitude to my parents and grandparents for supporting my academic pursuits and career aspirations that have brought me to where I am today. I feel endless gratitude for my mother, who modeled the honor of standing up for what you believe in, regardless of the danger and judgments involved in standing up for justice and democracy. I send endless gratitude to my caretaker and nanny, who demonstrated the power of the human spirit to overcome a life of trauma, grief, and chronic pain, while navigating institutional racism and sexism. Observing her medical experiences sparked my passion and lifelong mission to create a more humane, compassionate, effective, and accessible approach to healing trauma and chronic pain.

I feel deep gratitude for my lifelong love and partner for caring for and believing in me through my years of navigating pelvic and sexual pain, recovering from brain surgeries, and associated traumas.

I feel endless gratitude for my mentors, Gina Ogden and Charlie Curtis, for sharing their perspectives of the universe and offering a map and bridge of understanding between the physical, mental, emotional, and spiritual realms.

I wish to express gratitude for the mystical connections possible between us, as a human species on this abundant, diverse planet.

I send endless gratitude to the members of the International Pelvic Pain Society, as you have been my tribe, teachers, and friends.

Finally, I feel infinite gratitude for the opportunity to raise my child, who reminds me of the pure light and love that inhabits this world.

Thank you, all. Thank you.

Introducing Your Author and Chronic Pelvic Pain

My name is Alexandra Turgeon Milspaw. I am a licensed professional counselor in the state of Pennsylvania, an AASECT*-Certified sex therapist, and a certified 4-D Wheel practitioner. At the time of publication, I am serving as the Vice President of the 4-D Network and am the Director of Behavioral Health Services for Pelvic Rehabilitation Medicine.** I am certified in Mindfulness-Based Stress Reduction, Neuro-Linguistic Programming, and Consulting Hypnosis. I earned my PhD in Human Sexuality from Widener University and my Master's in Counseling Psychology and Human Services from Lehigh University. My Bachelor's degree is in Sociology and Anthropology with a minor in Women's Studies from Lehigh University, where I co-founded Break the Silence—a peer-education and 24-hour crisis line for gender violence.

My dissertation is entitled "Women's Histories and Their Experiences with Chronic Pelvic, Genital, and Sexual Pain," and I review some of the content and findings of my dissertation in this book. I have been studying this topic since the beginning of my career. I trained for five years with Robert Echenberg, MD, FACOG, who was one of the leading gynecologists and specialists in America at the time. Dr. Echenberg introduced me to the International Pelvic Pain Society (IPPS), for which I have served on the Board since 2020 and currently serve as Chair for their Clinical Foundations training program at their annual conferences.

Chronic pelvic pain (CPP) is a silent, multi-systemic disorder that affects more than 30 million American reproductive-aged women.

---

*American Association of Sexuality Educators, Counselors and Therapists
**A national, interdisciplinary physiatry clinic specializing in chronic pelvic pain.

CPP encompasses a web of disorders and involves the organs, nervous system, and musculoskeletal system, including, but not limited to, chronic pain and central sensitization, Vulvodynia/Vulvar Vestibulitis, Painful Bladder Syndrome (PBS), Irritable Bowel Syndrome (IBS), Endometriosis, neuropathies, Pelvic Floor Dysfunction (PFD), and Post-Traumatic Stress Disorder (PTSD).

Generalized chronic pain disorders affect 130 million women in the United States. Thirty million of those women experience chronic pelvic pain. Eighty to ninety percent of all patients suffering from CPP also suffer from some type of sexual pain disorder. It is estimated that 61 percent of women with CPP have not been diagnosed. CPP continues to be under-recognized, misdiagnosed, and unsuccessfully treated due to the lack of research and education of its complex pathology. Due to most doctors' lack of knowledge about CPP, patients undergo a plethora of tests and exploratory surgeries and procedures to seek the cause and treatment for their pelvic pain, which usually tends to complicate and intensify over time. The ineffective treatment of multiple surgeries detrimentally affects every aspect of a person's life. The guided exercises in this book will provide support in healing from all of the above.

I am very passionate about the pelvic and sexual pain population. One of my life's missions is to help bridge the gap between the medical and the psychological communities. I love collaborating with physical therapists and physicians. Intradisciplinary care is a critical aspect of treating chronic pelvic and sexual pain disorders. I worked in private practice for 12 years before joining the team at Pelvic Rehabilitation Medicine in October 2021. I'm in my dreamland when I'm collaborating with various healthcare providers all over the country.

Thank you for reading my book and dedicating time to empowering yourself with knowledge and skills that support your healing journey. It is my true honor and privilege to support you along your journey. Thank you for this opportunity. The light in me honors the light within you. May you allow the energy of well-being to flow through you like radiant health, vitality, and joy.

Chapter 1
There Is No Failure, Only Feedback

Many doctors and therapists will tell you that a healing protocol is not one size fits all. I work with many different people from different cultures, different geographical locations, different stages of healing, and different pain experiences. While you all share most of the same physiology, the way your brains react to the functioning of that physiology can vary. I'm certainly doing my best to speak to all of you, even though I don't know you.

I run a monthly all-gender support group for chronic pelvic pain (CPP) patients where they ask questions, meet each other, share stories and resources, and practice the exercises that I have included in this book. If you have the opportunity to join such a group, do consider it because increasing your social connections can raise serotonin levels, which help decrease inflammation.

This book is both educational and experiential. I teach you various facts about the brain, about the body, how pain is processed, and how trauma and stress affect that process, and ultimately I help you connect the dots of your life experience. I guide you through various exercises based in the study of Mindfulness-Based Cognitive Therapy, Neuro-Linguistic Programming, Energy Psychology, and Consulting Hypnosis. I encourage you to take notes about your experiences and practice what feels effective for you. I want you to take one step at a time and take each step when it feels right for you. How will you know when it's the right time? Know this: There is no failure, only feedback.

The most common feedback I receive from my clients is: (1) difficulty finding the time to practice these exercises, and (2) being overwhelmed with the information and all the resources. The key is to explore and discover the exercises that feel best for you. You don't have to do everything. The main idea is to support and calm the nervous system, and everything downstream from that will return to its natural state of homeostasis and well-being. Yes, I give you a lot of information in this book, and I want you to take it in stride. **Even if all you do for the next few minutes is pick up this book and read a random page or listen to a random exercise, that's enough! When you're ready and able to enjoy five minutes here and five minutes there to explore and discover more information about your experience, this will inspire you to create more opportunities to delve deeper into the process in a way that feels right for you.** You can follow the sample schedule on page 25) if that matches your style. As I describe in a moment, when we're trying to create healthy habits, there is a specific method that is important to consider. That method does not include any sense of force, or control, or shaming yourself into doing something (i.e., "shame on me for not doing more self-care today), or threatening yourself (i.e., "I won't ever heal if I don't do all of these exercises every day"). **Be gentle with yourself. Trust yourself.** Give yourself ample time to allow this information to soak in. Allow your mind, body, heart, and spirit to recalibrate as you continue to explore and discover the exercises that connect with you and guide you into that healing state of mind, body, heart, and spirit.

Who Should Be on Your Treatment Team

Below I list the best specialties to have on your "A" team, followed by a brief description of some of the treatments they can offer. A book could be written on every specialty! If I'm aware of a book by a specialist, I include it in the description.

▶ **Behavioral health**
  - Ideally offers: mindfulness, hypnosis, neurolinguistic programming, and autonomic nervous system regulation through somatic therapies and breath work
  - Book recommendation: *Sexual Healing* by Peter Levine, *The Heart and Soul of Sex* by Gina Ogden, and the book you're reading!

▶ **Acupuncture and Chinese medicine**
- Ideally offers: acupuncture, laser and light therapy, herbal remedies, homeopathy, and kinesiology (muscle testing) for Lyme, parasites, and other GI and immune disorders that may not be identified using Western Medicine tests
- Book recommendation: *The Essential Companion and Study Guide of Chinese Herbal Medicine* by Lisa Pilar Baas (lisabaashealingarts.com)

▶ **Yoga, Qi Gong, and Tai Chi**
- Ideally offers: gentle, mindful movement exercises that strengthen the posture muscles
- Book recommendation: *Iyingar Yoga for Motherhood* by Geeta Iyangar

▶ **Sound healing**
- Ideally offers: singing bowls, tuning forks, gongs, and other vibrational healing techniques
- Book recommendation: *Sound Healing* by Mitchell Gaynor, MD

▶ **Physiatry**
- Ideally offers: evaluation of whole-body movement and function, joint inflammation, nerve blocks, and other injections that can help heal the nerves in the hips and pelvis
- Book recommendation: *Chronic Pelvic Pain and Pelvic Dysfunctions: Assessment and Multidisciplinary Approach* edited by Alessandro Giammo and Antonella Biroli

▶ **Functional medicine**
- Ideally offers: holistic approach to evaluating the whole body and whole self
- Book recommendation: *Solving the Autoimmune Puzzle* by Keesha Ewers, MD

▶ **Pelvic floor physical therapy**
- Ideally offers: physical therapy to rehab the lower back, pelvis, hips, abdomen, diaphragm, posture correction, and whole-body

balancing to *relax and release* the tension and spasms in the pelvic floor muscles
- Book recommendations: *Heal Pelvic Pain* by Amy Stein; Mary Velicki's three-book healing series; *Pelvic Pain Explained* by Stephanie Prendergast

▶ **Gynecology**
- Ideally offers: evaluation of reproductive organs; rule out inflammatory and disease processes including endometriosis and fibroids
- Book recommendations: *Healing Painful Sex* by Deborah Coady, MD, and Nancy Fish, LCSW; *Silent Suffering* by Robert Echenberg, MD, and Susan Bilheimer

▶ **Nutrition**
- Ideally offers: support for anti-inflammatory diet, food substitutions and recipes, health coaching, and support for healthy lifestyle changes
- Book recommendations: any book by Jessica Drummond; nutrition courses by Monique Bogni at Pelvic Rehabilitation Medicine; *Painful Bladder Syndrome* by Philip Weeks

▶ **Gastrointestinal**
- Ideally offers: evaluation of gastrointestinal system, organ health and functional evaluation, rule out inflammatory and disease processes

▶ **Urology**
- Ideally offers: evaluation of bladder, kidneys, and prostate; rule out inflammatory and disease processes
- Book recommendation: *Headache in the Pelvis* by David Wise, MD

Chapter 2

What to Expect and How to Read This Book

The brain can only absorb so much information at once. Some people learn by listening (maybe you're listening to this right now on your audiobook app), some learn by reading, and some learn by watching. Everyone learns by doing. In this book, I try to provide all the above options. Throughout the book, you will see this symbol 🌳 indicating that you can learn more at my website, where you will find either an MP3 recording or a video of me demonstrating a specific exercise. To access the site, use the QR code in the box below. The more you experience the processes reviewed, the more likely you are to practice one of these exercises on your own. My goal is to empower you and help you understand how your body is capable of healing no matter how long you've been in pain or how severe it is. I seek to fill your toolbox of resources so you can feel resourceful. Surely, feeling resourceful is one of the most important resources you can allow. Even if you try just one exercise per month over the next six months, you're going to feel equipped to manage the pain and to continue the healing work on your own.

> Whenever you see this symbol 🌳, use this QR code to access more information at my website.

For now, read a section of the book, practice the exercise(s), then take a five-minute break before returning to the book. Take your time and allow yourself to fully integrate every experience you have and everything you learn.

Everything reviewed in this book is backed by research. I include an excerpt from my dissertation along with a comprehensive list of recommended books, websites, and other resources in the Appendices.

You never know when chronic pain is going to creep up in the nervous system. The oldest person with CPP I've worked with was 86 years old, and the youngest person I worked with was 9. I'll try to speak to the variations on how pelvic and sexual pain can affect us across the lifespan. CPP affects everyone in similar ways, but with different consequences.

It takes an average of five to seven years before an accurate diagnosis is provided by a CPP specialist. By then, the pain has created something called central sensitization, which will be discussed shortly. Whether you've had CPP for six months or 20 years, your brain and nervous system are always capable of reprogramming. This book will show you many ways to reprogram and retrain your brain and nervous system.

EXERCISE

On a scale from 1-10 (1 being low, 10 being high), what is your current level of belief and hope about your ability to heal? Write that here:

I'm going to ask you again at the end of this book. If I did my job, you'll finish this book at a 10.

For now, I wish that all of my hope for you becomes contagious. One thing I do say about the word "hope" is that hope in and of itself suggests a potential for the opposite of what you want, does it not? If I'm "hoping" to heal, that means I believe there is still a possibility of not healing. Rather, I prefer to use the word "trust." I want you to trust the process and trust that **your body is absolutely capable of healing**. I trust I can help you take in all the information you need to build this trust by understanding how your system works and how your system is capable of healing. But know this: **You already have all the resources you need.**

✏️▶ EXERCISE

Are you ready to heal? Circle Yes or No.

I invite you to set an intention to allow that to happen (now).

Healing is less about hope and more about trusting the process. You're here reading this, so clearly you already have a willingness to believe in your ability to change and heal. Thank you! I ask that you set that intention for yourself because that can be the foundation. Your intention is the fertilizer through which you're going to grow some of these new ideas in the garden of your mind. It is my hope that by the end of this book, you will understand the basic premise of how pain, trauma, and stress are processed within the brain and why healing the brain is a necessary component. I want you to understand the mind-body connection, how the brain changes with pain, and how understanding your individual brain map can help change your own perspective.

Within your personal experience of pain, particularly with pelvic and sexual pain, it often starts off with a bit of mystery and a lot of fear because of that mystery. Too many physicians do not understand CPP. Commonly, people have to go to more than five different physicians before they find an accurate diagnosis or find someone who knows what they're talking about, let alone someone who knows what the diagnosis is and understands how to guide you through the intradisciplinary healing process. If you're lucky to have found such a practitioner, this most likely took five to seven years, per the latest research. Sadly, I've never met someone with pelvic and sexual pain who wasn't told by at least one physician that they would just have to "get used to it." It should be illegal for a physician to say that healing is impossible. Obviously, if you have an amputation, you can't heal that (yet), but you can heal the pain of that amputation. (*The Graded Motor Imagery Handbook* by G. Lorimer Moseley, et al. is a good resource.)

As I've stated before,* in order to heal from chronic pain, it's important for you to understand the mind-body connection and understand how pain happens in order for you to gain a new perspective. That new perspective will guide the brain and the nervous system to respond differently. I seek to teach you to respond more calmly and with curiosity. I seek to empower you to know you have all the resources you need to manage the pain and speed up the healing process. Because, why not? I'm assuming you want to allow healing, am I right?

You can expect to learn at least three brain exercises that calm your nervous system and three new healthy behavioral habits that will ease your pelvic and sexual pain (three is a magic number, after all). In this book, I delve into a full intradisciplinary approach. For CPP, you want to treat it from all angles because of all the different organ systems and neuromuscular systems that are involved.

I'm going to teach you how to create at least three positive affirmations that feel true for you. I'm not simply talking about positive thinking, because positive thinking in and of itself doesn't work if you don't believe it. **You must *experience* a positive emotion if you want the thought to be powerful enough to affect your nervous system**. If there is too much of a belief gap between what you believe and what you say, you tend to slingshot back and feel even more anxious, depressed, and hopeless. Overall, I'm going to cover a lot of information. I want you to walk away with information, exercises, and resources you can utilize to manage the pain, manage life's stress, and relax your neuromuscular system and pelvic floor. Even if one doesn't work, you now have access to a large toolbox worth discovering in this book.

I'm going to delve into looking at the brain and how the brain changes with stress, trauma, and chronic pain. I'm going to discuss how brain maps and "pain maps" are created and what that means. Gaining a

---

* I like to repeat myself when I think it's important. ☺ You'll get to know me a bit more by the end of this book. Fun facts are everywhere!

bird's-eye view of what is happening in your system and what's happening when you experience pain helps you grab the reins on it a little bit more so you can turn the volume down on the intensity of the pain and suffering. It's important for you to learn how to steer the ship of your mind. You can't control the weather, but you can steer.* Always helpful. And yes, I'll be using a lot of metaphors throughout the book as well. Feel free to substitute them with your own!

Have you ever wondered, "What's happening in my brain when I'm thinking?" or "What's happening in my brain when I'm believing?" or "How does the frequency of my emotions affect the cellular patterns and the neural patterns of my neuromuscular system and my organs?" This is the science behind why you want to learn how to emotionally self-regulate, and how to utilize your emotions as a guidance system. If you're feeling a certain way, that means you're believing a certain thought. How can you change that thought pattern? How do you do that when it feels uncontrollable? My approach in this book goes well beyond Cognitive Behavioral Therapy (CBT). The more you understand the biology of your thoughts, beliefs, and emotions, the more you'll walk away with a clear understanding of why it's important to steer the ship. As you may have predicted, I'm going to discuss brainwaves and thought patterns and the biology of belief.

After that, I'll delve into mindfulness and compassionate curiosity. Looking at the evidence and the science behind the imagination, including sports psychology and how you use visualization and imagination to get the body to do what you want it to do. I'm going to review some research on how the power of imagination guides the body to heal faster.

Chapter 9 takes us into understanding how pain affects relationships and sexual health. Pelvic and sexual pain affects all aspects of life and sexuality, including how you relate and interact with others.

Chapter 10 reviews light therapy and sound therapy. I'll review the science behind red, infrared, and near infrared light and how it heals connective tissue, nerves, neural connections, and muscle cells.

---

* "Steer" is a great song by Missy Higgins.

I'm going to give you enough information to help you understand, and therefore motivate you to do some of these exercises daily. I know that when I was first learning meridian tapping—a bilateral stimulation exercise—I wished I knew the science behind it. In hindsight, I think that would have given me more motivation to practice it. I want to give you a foundation of knowledge and motivate you. I'm also going to talk about how to shift the trauma response in your body with bilateral stimulation. Are you excited to learn this?

DID YOU KNOW?

When you're in fight-or-flight mode, the left and right hemispheres of your brain are not communicating effectively. Both sides of the brain need to communicate clearly in order to help process and file away the events and the stress that you're experiencing. Bilateral stimulation exercises create this bridge by waking up the left and right hemispheres of your brain through stimulation of the left and right sides of your body via visual, auditory, or kinesthetic stimulation. Bilateral stimulation helps create a "bridge" between the left and right hemispheres through moving your eyes back and forth (visual), hearing different sounds in each ear using headphones (auditory), or tapping on both sides of your body (kinesthetic). This improves activity, communication, and circulation in your brain. You need your brain to heal and return to functioning in a balanced way in order to your nervous system to its natural state of well-being.

The bilateral stimulation practice is absolutely key (see "Emotional Freedom Techniques" on page 102). Once you do that, then we're able to utilize the mindfulness-based cognitive therapy (MBCT) to update the software. **We're healing the hardware, and then we're going to update the software.**

Basic talk therapy and CBT techniques try to update the software before updating the hardware, and the brain is not able to "click save" for a long time. Many people don't find that helpful in the long term. There is a 65 percent relapse rate for chronic pain and trauma patients within six months if they only practice CBT. When you start with healing the brain and getting the hemispheres of the brain to communicate the way you need them to, it's a lot more effective, efficient, and sustainable. When you add bilateral stimulation and mindfulness, relapse decreases to 15 to 25 percent.

Getting Ready to Learn

I recommend having a special healing notebook so you can keep all of the notes that you take while reading this book and practicing these exercises together in one place. This enables you to be able to review it more easily. Hopefully you come with an open mind and you're curious. Certainly, you're here, so you already have a bit of an open mind. What you put into this process is what you're going to get out of it.

Healing is not a linear process. Healing is not about achieving specific goals. Healing is a yearning to become your best self—your greatest self. Healing is about creating deep emotional change, self-actualization—a deep belief in yourself—and from there, you notice yourself making different choices, which lead to changes and momentum toward your goals of healing like never before. Healing is a lifestyle.

If you're feeling super ambitious, three workbooks are useful to have on your shelves. Some of the exercises I am going to teach you are inspired by these authors and researchers. The first is *Unlearn Your Pain*, coauthored by Dr. Howard Schubiner, who works very closely with Dr. John Sarno, the author of *The Mindbody Prescription*. Their work demonstrates one end of the spectrum, which states that the brain fully and completely can heal your pain. However, I find that with pelvic and sexual pain, the intradisciplinary approach is often necessary. Nevertheless, the mind and brain are powerful forces that should not be underestimated.

I've seen and experienced miraculous healing over the past 20 years, some of which I will share with you throughout this book. Case studies can be inspiring, more so than dry research, which is why I include these stories in this book. Similar case studies can be found in Dr. Lissa Rankin's *The Fear Cure* and *Mind over Medicine* books. Centuries of case studies within the field of hypnosis and psychoneuroimmunology demonstrate the power of the mind over the body. Unfortunately, these case studies have not yet made it into the curriculum of medical and psychology training programs. I will share some of those incredible statistics and stories with you in hopes that they inspire you in the same way that they inspire me.

Another workbook I recommend is *The Mindful Way Workbook* by Segal, et al. This workbook reviews some of the mindfulness-based stress-reduction exercises and comes with guided meditations. The resources you have access to through this book, along with my YouTube channel ("Dr. Alex Milspaw" at www.youtube.com/dralexmilspaw) provide similar experiences. 🌲

Finally, *The Explain Pain Handbook: Protectometer* is a handbook by Lorimer Moseley and David Butler. These two researchers and practitioners have led the world in pain research over the past 20 years, and their phenomenal handbook guides you through pain education and how to think differently about the pain. I will review some of their work in later chapters.

My presupposition to all of this is that you need to heal the organ of the brain in order for any of this information be able to click save. Nevertheless, these three great workbooks can be useful if you're wanting to do all of the above.

Supplements I Recommend Starting Now

I will discuss the importance of healing the gastrointestinal (GI) system in order to heal the brain. The following supplements do wonders, so I want to highlight and recommend starting these immediately: Lionsmane mushroom, turkey tail mushroom, magnesium, and EnteroMend®.

Lionsmane mushroom heals neurological damage both in the brain and in the peripheral nerves. If you experience nerve pain and brain fog, Lionsmane is useful to get started on right away. Most clients I work with report feeling a higher sense of mental clarity and reduced nerve-burning sensations after a month of taking this supplement.

Turkey tail mushroom is useful for reducing systemic inflammation. If you have endometriosis or any other autoimmune dysregulation such as multiple sclerosis, Sjogren's, Lyme, Hashimoto's, lupus, or related joint pain and/or GI inflammation, turkey tail mushroom is really going to help calm that down. More information on the healing qualities of mushrooms can be found in the documentary "Fantastik Fungi" available on Netflix and at Paul Stamet's website. Please see the longer list of resources in Appendix E.

Magnesium is great for improving GI function as well as neuromuscular relaxation and sleep. Some CPP specialists recommend Calm® powder, which is magnesium carbonate. This has been demonstrated in the research to have increased absorption rates. I tend to recommend magnesium oxide because it can be more gentle on GI function while providing optimal neuromuscular relaxation. However, if you experience severe constipation, Calm® powder may be more effective for you. If you're already on magnesium, stick with what you currently take. As always, **please follow your physician's guidance for any vitamins and supplements**. You do not want to double up on multiple magnesium types because you can take too much. I recommend starting at 250 milligrams and increasing from there as needed, with a maximum of 1,000 milligrams. Always start low and slow with any new medications, vitamins, and supplements. Start one at a time so you can know which one is causing any change or improvements.

EnteroMend® (I recommend the Health Concerns brand) is a digestive enzyme that will significantly decrease the inflammatory response of whatever it is that you're eating. If you're not ready to do a full diet cleanse to really help heal the GI system, EnteroMend®, magnesium, and turkey tail mushroom will be a great start to regulating GI function. The GI system is a main trigger for pelvic floor muscle spasms and pelvic nerve sensitivity. GI function also strongly influences brain function. If you experience chronic constipation, you may tend to have depression-related symptoms. If you experience diarrhea or loose bowels, you may tend to have more anxiety-related symptoms. If you experience Irritable Bowel Syndrome (IBS) where function alternates between constipation and diarrhea, you may tend to have more mood fluctuations. Brain health is highly connected with GI health.

Tiny Tweaks Lead to Big Changes—Begin Creating Healthy Habits Now!

Right now, I invite you to create special time every day, ideally twice a day, to devote to exploring and practicing the exercises included in this book. It is ideal to build up to at least 20 minutes a day because the majority of research on mindfulness and meditation is built on a consecutive 20-minute practice. However, in my professional and personal experience, practice can also be effective if you scatter this time throughout the day, i.e., 10 minutes in the morning, at lunch, and in the evening. I recommend starting with five minutes in the morning and five minutes in the evening and build on that each week. See the sample schedule on page 25.

Overall, I want you to set intentions for yourself on a regular basis. Maybe you set your intention to read one chapter a week. Maybe your intention is to practice one exercise every day after a meal. Setting intentions cannot be underestimated. Take a moment to do that now.

◀▶ EXERCISE

I set an intention to
(read/practice/think) every day at   :   PM/AM
for the next week.

Think about how you want to reward yourself each week for setting these intentions and following through. The more you can stay in that habit of self-care utilizing an exercise that's very effective for you, the easier it is to thread it into your everyday lifestyle.

TAKE THINGS AT YOUR OWN PACE

For effective, efficient brain healing to begin, I recommend starting with the supplements I mentioned earlier and the bilateral stimulation of either Emotional Freedom Techniques or audio music available by Jeffrey Thompson or hemi-sync.com. I am going to talk about bilateral stimulation in more detail a little later. (See page 23.) Bilateral stimulation is a huge component in helping heal your brain hemispheres so they communicate, process, and file away information accurately and effectively.

There are three Rs to creating healthy habits: routine, reminder, and reward.

▶ **Routine:** Practice something at the same time every day. Routines are extremely effective in calming the nervous system. When you have a history of trauma, stress, and chronic pain, *predictability* is soothing to the system. Routines create predictability.

▶ **Reminder:** Set a reminder on your phone or ask a friend or a partner to practice this with you. I know I am more likely to go on a walk if my neighbor is waiting for me outside. When you have someone to practice healthy habits with, you are more likely to follow through on your intentions.

▶ **Reward:** Create a reward for yourself for the small and big accomplishments. A reward can certainly be the benefit of practicing the self-care exercise, such as feeling calm after tapping (EFT). Rewarding yourself in other ways is important in helping your brain click save. Some ideas of rewards for practicing a week of daily self-care include visiting your favorite restaurant, taking a long bath with essential oils and good music, or watching your favorite movie.

THINGS TO REMEMBER WHEN CREATING HEALTHY HABITS

All things in nature operate
on a rhythm of well-being.

Consistency is more important
than duration.

If you don't like the story, rewrite it.

There is no failure, only feedback.

Do you want to be right, or do
you want to be happy?

Focus on what you want for at least 17
seconds. BOOM! You've created neurons.

Thriving is what is natural to you.

The Dynamic Three Vs for Achieving Goals*

1. **Verbalize:** We constantly verbalize with words, either talking to others or to ourselves. The words we use determine our lives and achievements. Words like: "I am," "I can," and "I will" in our positive goal statements can have really great results. Write down your ideas, using these terms. You'll be surprised at the almost explosive empowering effect this has on feelings of self-esteem, confidence, capability, competence, and in fact, on every aspect of your energy and of your life. French pharmacist Emile Coué worked miracles with sick, lame, disenfranchised French peasants by teaching them to say, "Every day, in every way, I am getting better and better." Now you can create your own miracles.

2. **Visualize:** We all have created in our minds some sort of mental image of ourselves and of exactly what we can do, and we are running that mental movie of ourselves in our heads all the time. Decide what kind of person you want to become and what you want to accomplish and develop a clear-cut mental picture. Write down a vivid description, using your senses of seeing and hearing and feeling, as to how you may need to change, and begin right now to verbalize and visualize it as your virtual reality.

3. **Vitalize:** We spend our lives acting out the mental pictures of ourselves that we have made. To vitalize means to add life to, to animate, to develop vigor, and to bring into being. So, we add emotions and life to our goals by our actions. And that's just exactly what we need to do: add emotions to put our words and pictures into action by embodying and acting out our goals with energy and enthusiasm. Each day write down the actions you are taking to make your dreams come true. And enjoy what is happening to and for you.

---

* Adapted by N.S. Curtis © 2012 NLP Training Class, borrowed from Bob Conklin, Ego-Bionics

TINY TWEAKS

One of my favorite routines: Upon waking in the morning, I take three deep breaths and feel gratitude for having another day to continue creating the life that I love. That may be my only practice for the day. Maybe I want to take three deep breaths before I fall asleep and feel gratitude for three things that I experienced during my day. I enjoy feeling gratitude for all that was good in the day so I feel content and sleep content.

It may seem too subtle and easy, but again, sometimes these tiny tweaks can really lead to significant changes when you look at how the brain and the nervous system function.

EXERCISE

Create your three Rs now. Set a time and a reminder and choose the reward for this week.

Routine:

Reminder:

Reward:

TIP

Start practicing some of these techniques at the same time you are doing something else that is already part of your daily routine. For instance, you already brush your teeth every day twice a day, so perhaps when you're brushing your teeth, that's when you're really tuning in and practicing mindfulness. Maybe that's when you're saying the mantra to yourself: "I'm allowing my body to heal."

If you piggyback your self-care time with something that you are already doing, you can ensure that you maintain the routine. The brain is more likely to practice something that creates a reward. Sometimes the exercise itself will be the reward, due to engaging the parasympathetic nervous system (the calm, restorative state of the nervous system), and often this causes the brain to create its own "bliss" hormones. For example, many of the exercises that you will learn in this book can boost dopamine (the happy neurochemical), oxytocin (the bonding hormone), and the literal "bliss" molecule called "anandamide."*

Sample Daily Routine for Systemic Healing

Remember, the main focus is to calm your nervous system by increasing safety, security, and trust. Your mind is learning to believe your body will respond to your interventions. (The mind needs three to five rewarding experiences to stop anticipating the painful response.) Your

---

* Check out *Bliss Brain* by Dawson Church.

body is learning to believe your mind will listen when it has something to say. (It needs to know that you're going to listen when it tells you you're in pain, versus pushing through the pain.)

Follow the pyramid process:

I.   Awareness: What are you aware of?

II.   Breath control: Does practicing breath work help?
   a. If no, go to bilateral stimulation
   b. If yes, go to body flow

III.   Bilateral stimulation: Listen to Jeffrey Thompson's music, sway back and forth, and/or practice Emotional Freedom Techniques until your nervous system calms down and you're able to practice breath work.
   a. Jeffrey Thompson: www.scientificsounds.com – also on Spotify, Amazon, and iTunes
   b. Emotional Freedom Techniques: www.thetappingsolution.com and YouTube

IV.   Body flow: Is your body able to move in a fluid, flowing way? Are you able to sway like a willow tree blowing in the breeze?
   a. If yes, you're ready to work on the mental quadrant.
   b. If no, practice Qi Gong, Tai Chi, or dance! Practice moving your body in a fluid way until it feels comfortable.

V.   Mental quadrant: observing thoughts, beliefs, inner commentary
   a. Mindful journaling #1–20, thought labels on odd numbers and physical sensations on even numbers (See page 98.)
   b. Rational Emotive Behavioral Therapy (REBT) (See worksheet on page 148.)
   c. Rewriting your narrative and how you tell your story of who you are and what's possible for you

    d. Free-writing journaling—dumping your thoughts onto paper without trying to make "rational" sense or even sentences, just letting it all out

    e. Are you able to do any of these exercises and feel calm?

       i. If no, go back to bilateral stimulation. Utilize EFT or Dr. Thompson's music to help you process the mental quadrant's noise that is keeping your brain "stuck."

      ii. If yes, wonderful! You've created a new mindset and perspective for yourself. Keep practicing—this is a lifelong skill and exercise to rethink your assumptions, beliefs, and thoughts.

"If you think time will change your ways, don't wait too long."

—Madeline Pereoux

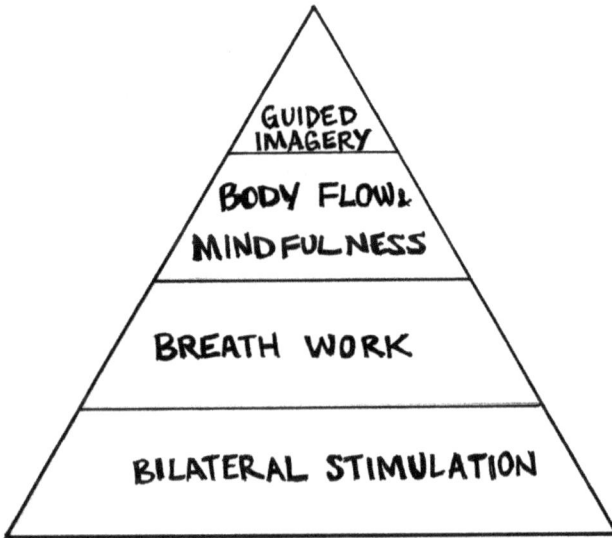

10-MINUTE MORNING RITUAL
TO FEEL GOOD*

1. Smile for one minute. Doing it in front of the mirror is even better.

2. Meditate on something positive for five minutes (or more, if you have the extra time).

3. Use virtual reality: Visualize something you desire, using all of your senses to achieve vibrational alignment for the last four minutes.

4. Keep happy, prosperous thoughts uppermost in your mind all day. Try the Place Mat Exercise** when you can.

5. Remember: We each create our own reality, for better or worse, by the thoughts we entertain in our minds all day.

Sample Daily Schedule

Waking Up
- Think and feel gratitude for another day to live and heal.
- Set an intention for the day (one big or three small intentions).

Rising for the Day
- Start your day with a cup of hot/warm water—even add a few drops of fresh lemon to help cleanse the lymphatic system and GI system and prepare it for the day's meals
- Practice Qi Gong for 10 to 20 minutes.

---

* Adapted by Nancy Curtis © 2012, NLP Training Class, Reprinted with permission.

** Place Mat Exercise: Create a place mat that you can use daily that has images and words to remind you of your goal and what healing looks like and feels like for you.

- Do dry brushing before your shower. (Search for videos on You-Tube.)
- Sing in the shower for breath work and sound healing.
- Do a five-senses check-in during the shower– "4D Mindful I Spy" at my website 🌳
  - What do you see? Smell? Hear? Taste? Feel?
- Brush your teeth with your non-dominant hand. (This engages your brain to pay attention to what you're doing and how you're doing it!)
- Take Vitamin D 5000 IU and mushroom supplements (turkey tail, lionsmane, reishi)

Mealtimes

- Eat one bite mindfully (see the Raisin Exercise on page 277).
- Make eye contact with someone you're sharing a meal with and feel gratitude and love for their company. (And if they cooked it for you, say thank you and mean it.)
- Say to yourself, "Everything I put into my body turns to health and happiness," no matter what you're eating.
- Take an EnteroMend® digestive enzyme if you're eating dairy, gluten, sugar, or soy.
- Play "I spy" with all five senses (see the shower exercise above).
- Check-in with your intentions that you set that morning; reflect, adjust, refresh as needed.

30 Minutes before Bedtime

- Wear blue light-blocking glasses or turn that mode on your TV and phone/tablet. (This allows your brain to start creating its own melatonin for deeper sleep.)
- Do restorative yoga poses with your head supported and/or Qi Gong or Tai Chi.
- Drink a cup of kava tea, which is very relaxing and sedating for neuromuscular body and mind.
- Set an intention for a deep, restorative sleep.
- Take 250 to 500 milligrams of magnesium oxide.
- Do meditation and bilateral stimulation.

- Listen to Jeffrey Thompson music or a meditation.
- Utilize light therapy while listening to a 10 to 20 minute meditation on my website 🌲 such as the "Ecomeditation.mp3" or "physical wellbeing.mp3" or the "chakra balancing with the breath.mp3" or any others you enjoy.
- Watch an episode of *Headspace* on Netflix.

Sample Six-week Progression of Healing Activities

Week 1

- 10 minutes per day of curiosity and intention
  - 60 seconds every hour, or
  - 5 minutes of practice in the AM and PM
- Explore and create your brain map utilizing the 4-D Wheel (See page 31.)
- 4D Mindful I Spy 🌲
- Extra: Identify a song that inspires you.

Week 2

- 15 minutes per day of curiosity and practice
  - 5 minutes AM, noon, and PM
- Extra: Write a letter to your past/younger self. What do you wish you knew back then that you know and understand now?

Week 3

- 20 minutes per day of curiosity and practice
  - 5 minutes AM, 5 minutes noon, and 10 minutes PM
- Create your "jar of ideas" for coping with DIMs and increasing SIMs. (See page 118.)
- Journal about DIMs and SIMs, then tap on them to help your brain neutralize unhelpful thoughts and beliefs.
- Extra: Have a conversation/dialogue with your body.

Week 4

- 25 minutes per day of curiosity and practice
  - 10 minutes AM, 5 minutes noon, and 10 minutes PM

- Mindful eating
- Extra: Write a letter to your present self from your future, healed self.

Week 5

- 30 minutes per day of curiosity and practice
  - 10 minutes AM, 10 minutes noon, 10 minutes PM
- Watch the "Anatomy of trust" video by Brené Brown, PhD, at www.brenebrown.com.
- Do the "How to connect with anyone" video eye-gazing exercise. (Search for it on YouTube.)
- Place cue cards on the dinner table to do with family and friends. (See the "Planting Seeds of Love" cue cards on page 226.)
- Practice changing "should" to "wish" in conversations that include feedback.
- Watch "The 4 Horsemen" video by John Gottman, at: www.gottman.com; recognize and manage criticism, defensiveness, contempt, and stonewalling in relationships.

Week 6

- 30 to 60 minutes per day of curiosity and practice
  - 20 minutes AM, noon, and PM
- Place a timer on your Wi-Fi router to your limit exposure to electromagnetic fields (EMF).
- Write a letter to your present self from your future self.
- Set intentions for the next three weeks to review what you've learned and continue the great progress you've started!
- Join a support groups to continue practicing and sharing your experiences with others.

Super-Learning

The secret to super-learning is to relax the system before absorbing new information. One thing you know about the autonomic nervous system (ANS) is that when you are in pain, you are in fight-or-flight mode. When you're in fight-or- flight mode, the only part of the ANS you can gain control over is your breath. You can't think really hard and control your heart rate or your metabolism or your pupil dilation or your hormones or your sweat glands. You can't consciously control any part of the ANS except for your breath. That's when you utilize the breath and lengthen the exhalation. When you lengthen the exhalation, you can pull the entire ANS with you, and that's why it can be so effective.

If you have any dysautonomia, or if you've had autonomic dysregulation for a long time, sometimes the breath work in and of itself is not going to be as effective for you initially. Nevertheless, know that with practice and with bringing in vibration or humming, which activates the vagus nerve, you can deepen the relaxation response.

BREATHE LIKE A BEE

This breathing exercise is called the Bumblebee Breath. You're going to inhale completely through the nose, then allow the exhalation to last as long as possible as you hum like a bee. This can also be done with any vowel sound that feels good for you (i.e., ah, ee, eye, oh, oo). *Note:* There are more oxygen receptors in the back of the nasal cavity so that's why breathing in through the nose increases oxygen in the brain a lot faster than breathing in through the mouth.

If you're new to breathing exercises, you can feel a little lightheaded for this reason. Repeat this five times. Take a moment to notice and note how this exercise made you feel.

Therefore, let's take a moment now to practice some breath work and invite the system to enter into a calm, receptive state of mind. You can practice any of the breathing exercises I have described in Appendix B or you can practice the exercise in the colored box on the next page.

A Few Notes on How to Take Notes

If you only read or listen to information, you tend to retain about 10 to 15 percent of the information. If you're taking notes, retention jumps to 60 to 70 percent.

If you relax and move your body throughout the process of learning, which is what I try to loop in throughout this book, you're going to retain close to all of it. That's one of the main reasons why this book includes experiential exercises. I want to help your system relax. I want to help your body move. I want to really help your brain get the most out of your time in reading or listening to this book.

As often as you remember:
- Write down your experiences and things that stand out to you.
- Write down your questions as you go along.
- Draw pictures and representations of ideas and concepts.
  For example, I'll talk about the garden of the mind. Perhaps you want to draw your own little garden and the metaphorical plants you want to plant in your garden. (See page 142.) Maybe you even identify the "weeds" or "invasive plants" (negative thoughts, unhelpful beliefs) that need to be pulled. Pictures and pictorial representations (metaphors and symbolism) of the concepts that stand out to you can be really powerful for you. I'm going to take you through various exercises to demonstrate that.
- Finally, keep all of your notes in one place so you can reference them later. This will help you as you move forward.

Setting Intentions with the 4-D Wheel

Now, let's get started with setting more specific intentions. I'm going to talk you through a process utilizing the 4-D Wheel of Sexual Experience created by Gina Ogden, PhD. (See the worksheet and more information in Appendix C.) The 4-D Wheel is useful for a mindful check-in with yourself and also for setting intentions. *I recommend walking the 4-D Wheel on a daily basis to help you practice mindfulness, set intentions, dialogue with your body, and discover the layers of your experience to focus on when practicing the brain exercises taught throughout this book.*

The 4-D Wheel

- The template is ancient and universal.
- You will explore the deepest truths of your sexual stories: body, mind, heart, and spirit.
- The work is safe, moving, collaborative, fun, and often surprising.
- You can use it immediately.

The Four-Dimensional Wheel approach to body, mind, heart, and spirit is an embodied practice. It springs from spiritual principles that honor all people, all diversity, all life. It is grounded in systems theory and sex survey research, and it has developed through decades of clinical practice. Its healing effects are often extraordinary; they are affirmed by findings of contemporary neuroscience.

EXERCISE

In your notebook, draw the 4-D Wheel with four quadrants and the center, as shown below.

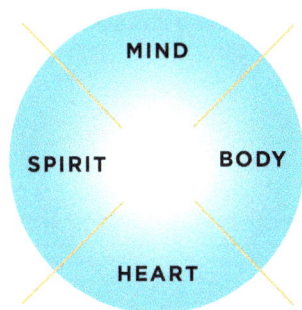

4-D NETWORK
Healing Body, Mind, Heart, & Spirit

Understanding the Quadrants

Mind

The mind quadrant stands for the mental story, the mental narrative, aka "the monkey mind." What are your thoughts? What are your beliefs? What do you know? What don't you know? What's happening in your mind?

Body

The body quadrant is the physical story, the physical sensations, the physical experiences. Where do you sense pain, tension, resistance? Where do you sense pleasure, relaxation, flow? Where is there function? Where is there dysfunction? When you're thinking a specific thought, where do you feel your body reacting? For example, do you feel your throat contract? Do you feel a ball of anxiety in your chest? Do you feel your stomach turn? You feel your emotions through physical sensations. *Note:* Trauma teaches the body to shut down emotional responses that feel overwhelming and unsafe, and so the body tries to release this energy through physical manifestations.

Heart

The heart quadrant is the emotional story. What emotions are you feeling? Emotions include: excitement, hope, doubt, guilt, shame, anxiety, worry, overwhelm, joy, eagerness. Notice all of the emotions that feel present for you. Emotions are e-motions = energy in motion. All emotions are energetic responses (electromagnetic frequencies that can be measured) to your thoughts and surroundings. What's your emotional story?

Spirit

The spirit quadrant is the experience of connection and disconnection. This is the quadrant of all relationships and whether you feel connected or disconnected to yourself, your partner(s), your friends, your social life, your family, and to a higher power, depending on your belief system. Pain is a common trigger for existential crises depending on your cultural, ethnic, and religious backgrounds. (See *The Pain Chronicles* by Melanie Thernstrom for a more detailed review of historical and religious teachings on the meaning of pain.) The spirit quadrant is where you explore your relationships, memories, and interactive experiences. The spirit quadrant is where you can identify feeling grounded or feeling dissociated.*

Each quadrant has a light side and a shadow side. All feedback is useful. All feedback is important. Instead of labeling something "positive" or "negative," categorize it in the light side or the shadow side. Whatever *no longer* serves your highest good—anything you want to release from your experience—goes into the shadow side. Whatever serves your highest good—anything you want to invite into your experience—goes into the light side.

First, I'm going to talk you through how to utilize the 4-D Wheel with setting intentions and answering, "What does healing look like?" Then I will demonstrate how to utilize the 4-D Wheel as a map for meditation and mindful check-ins with yourself. Finally, I will demonstrate how to utilize the 4-D Wheel to go deeper into your understanding of your experience so you can **connect the dots of your experience and create lasting change.** The 4-D Wheel is the main map you can utilize throughout your life to create understanding and intentions that are comprehensive and fulfilling.

EXAMPLE OF SETTING INTENTIONS WITH THE 4-D WHEEL

Mind
Shadow: "My doctor said get used to it."—"I won't get better."
Light: "Healing is possible."

---

*Dissociation is a common reaction to trauma and pain. I provide scripts of exercises in Appendix C to support those of you who experience dissociation and find it difficult to listen to a guided exercise.

Body
Shadow: Nerve pain
Light: Relaxation and pleasure

Heart
Shadow: Shame, fear
Light: Hope, joy

Spirit
Shadow: Disconnect from my body, my authentic self, my partner
Light: Connection, trust, feeling grounded and peaceful, more time with friends

What do you want to let go of or release from your experience? Place that in the shadow side. What do you want to invite in or strengthen? Place that in the light side.

Create Your Intentions Using the 4-D Wheel

Every time you get to a new chapter in this book, utilize the 4-D Wheel to check in with yourself. This is a mindfulness exercise as well as a powerful tool for setting intentions and remembering in what direction you want to move. You can follow along with my guided meditations around the 4-D Wheel on the book's webpage. 🌳

EXERCISE

Use an enlarged image of the 4-D Wheel for a mindful check-in:

- Place the large 4-D Wheel image on the floor and step into it.

- Start in the mind quadrant. What are you thinking?

- Step into the body quadrant. What physical sensations are you aware of? Scan your whole body.

- Step into the heart quadrant. What are you feeling?

- Step into the spirit quadrant. What images and relationships come to mind? Are you feeling connected or disconnected? Are you feeling more dissociated or grounded?

Walk the Wheel and Go Deeper

Instead of following the sequence in the exercise above, stand next to the quadrant you wish to start on. Think about one of your intentions. As you focus on the aspect of that intention within that quadrant (i.e., the pain within the Body quadrant), what else do you notice *in this moment* that's happening in your body? What are the other sensations that you experience when you tune into what you want to release or invite in? Do you become aware of an emotion, memory, relationship, or thought when you are focused on those sensations? When you do, move to that quadrant and notice what you become aware of. When you move to a different quadrant, move in a clockwise direction around the 4-D Wheel. Even if you are in the Body quadrant and you want to move to the Mind quadrant, walk all the way around the 4-D Wheel. This creates, literally and energetically, a spiral of movement, that leads you into the center of the 4-D Wheel, where you have those "a-ha" moments of insight, connection, and integration. Continue this process for as long as you desire, noting all of the connections that you may not have noticed or acknowledged before. Take a moment to write down what stood out to you about that process. Notice how when you walk around the 4-D Wheel, this helps you connect with and observe the various aspects of your experience (past, present, and future) you may not have noticed before. As you walk the 4-D Wheel, this helps your mind shift perspective and go deeper into your experience.

Acceptance: What It Is and What It Is NOT

When navigating chronic pain and trauma, many people can have an aversion to the word "acceptance," so here is a different definition of what acceptance means. When you're confronted by life or life events, you have three main options: (1) turn a blind eye and ignore the obvious; (2) stay, struggle, and complain; (3) accept it and face up to the fact that there is a problem. What do you learn from ignoring the obvious? When you ignore the problem, you encourage a belief of being helpless and a sense of not being responsible. You create an external locus of control—a belief that controlling the situation is outside of you, rather than inside of you. This does not breed resourcefulness. With CPP, you're likely waiting a long time to find a provider who knows what's going on, and when you find one, it can take months to get an appointment. This creates a delay in healing. What do you learn from complaining or suffering? You learn that you don't have a choice, that you're a victim of circumstance, that no one cares and nothing will change. Comparatively, when you move into a place of acceptance, it helps you figure out where you are on the map. If I'm driving to a new destination, I have to first accept where I am in order to be able to have a clear idea of how I am going to get from where I am. That's why the 4-D Wheel encourages you to answer, "What does healing look like?" You need to have a destination.

"Acceptance provides a standpoint before a change in action. Acceptance makes room for unlimited possibility and an opportunity to make the best and find the good in anything. [...] When you accept things that you cannot change you

**free yourself up to focus on things that you can.
When you know that you can make a difference,
you experience self-empowerment. When you are
empowered, you have the will, motivation, and
stamina to achieve your goals. With beliefs like that
I guess you could succeed at anything you want!"**
—Maya Mendoza, author of
The Hidden Power of Emotional Intuition

Where are you on the map? Earlier, you walked the 4-D Wheel to explore the current status of your body, heart, spirit, and mind, and the connections between them. Acceptance of where you are can start with an awareness of your experience.

I know a path is possible for every single person who is reading this book. Sometimes, acceptance starts with an accurate diagnosis. Useful components of having an accurate diagnosis are: (1) knowing you're not alone (if the diagnosis exists, clearly there's a large population of folks who experience the same thing); (2) a starting point for treatment. When you know that you have a toolbox to choose from, it helps change the fear response. Think of first responders, such as firefighters. They accept that they're walking into fire, and they accept that it's a very dangerous experience, but they put their trust in their training and in the resources that they've gained. They are less afraid of the fire because they know what to do when they're in that situation.

That's what I want for you. I want you to no longer fear the pain. Instead, I want you to feel resourceful. When you feel the pain, I want your mind to remember what you can do to help alleviate it. **Write this down and say it out loud: "I have all the resources I need."** This is one of the most powerful phrases for the subconscious mind. You may not feel that way right now, but you will. Self-empowerment helps create a calmer nervous system.

P = Please
A = Ask
I = Invite
N = Nurture

An acronym for pain is "please ask, invite, and nurture." Using mindfulness, I'm going to teach you how to ask your body what it needs, invite yourself to take a break and to tune in, and to nurture the whole self—mind, body, heart, and spirit. Remember walking the 4-D Wheel and asking each part what it was experiencing, wanting, needing? During this process, you're also inviting your body to share a dialogue with you—to tell you what your body is holding onto. You can ask your body questions such as:

- What are you trying to protect me from?
- What are you remembering?
- What are you needing?
- What are you desiring?
- How can I nurture you?

How you nurture all aspects of yourself affects your experience of pain.

I want you to identify two objects: (1) one object that represents everything that you're wanting to release from your experience, and (2) one object that represents everything you want to invite in and strengthen. As they say, pictures speak a thousand words. An intentional action you can do with these objects is to place the first object near a window. This represents your intention to allow the wind to carry away all that no longer serves your highest good. Place the second object near the front door. This represents your intention to allow all that serves your highest good to enter into your life. These objects can be anything as long as they represent what's important to you. Some examples that I've observed in the past include: a dilator that represented the sexual pain and feelings of shame; a heart-shaped pillow that represented love and acceptance and healthy relationships; a veil that represented feeling trapped in an unhappy marriage; a picture of a plane that represented the ability to travel and feel free.

EXERCISE

I want you to make a list of at least five times you have succeeded at learning something new. Then, next to each item you've listed, write down how that skill has benefited your life.

Here are some examples:

- Learned to read—helped me learn new things and feel smarter

- Learned to walk—helped me get around more easily and faster

- Learned to talk—helped me communicate my needs

- Learned to drive—gave me more freedom and helped me be able to escape the stress of my home and feel independent as a teenager

- Learned to ride a bike—gave me more freedom and helped me get to my friend's house faster

Take a moment to make your list now. Now, I want you to write at the bottom of this list:

"I am capable of learning new skills that benefit my life."

Anytime any part of going through this book is feeling too difficult or overwhelming, or if you get lost in that monkey mind of "I'm not good at this," or "I can't," or "I'm so overwhelmed," or "My brain feels completely full," or "I don't know if I could learn anything," I want you to review this evidence and read this statement. Writing it down helps the brain click save. You may even want to decorate it in your notebook. Doodling helps the brain! Children are now allowed to doodle more often in school because the research is pretty clear on how it helps the brain click save. When you're going through your notes, I want some of these things to stand out. Say this to yourself again: "I'm capable of learning new skills that benefit my life."

Here's something else that I want you to write down:

"There is no failure, only feedback."

Big corporations are finally catching on to that. You may have been taught to avoid failure at all costs. You may have been taught so much shame around failure. Is that true for you? Nevertheless, thanks to the leaders of Google and Amazon and others, we now know that embracing failure, and even rewarding failure, increases learning and success. When failure is not feared, people tend to try harder and take more risks, and they always learn more.

Therefore, with any of the exercises you learn in this book, remember, there is no failure, only feedback! You can't fail at a breathing exercise. You can't fail at mindfulness. I'm going to teach you how to tune into the feedback so you can learn from every experience and every practice. For example, if your brain is unable to focus on a visualization, the feedback is that you need to calm the autonomic nervous system (ANS) first through bilateral stimulation and breathwork.

The next thing you're going to write down in your notebook is the pyramid process. This is also found in the Sample Daily Routine for Systemic Healing on page 25. Draw this image:

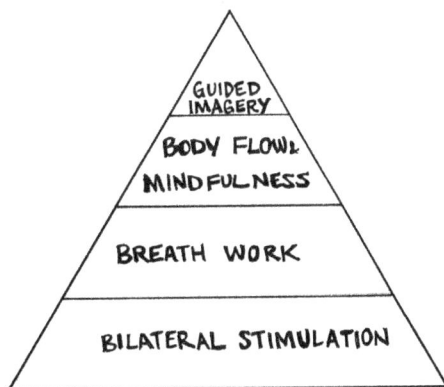

The most powerful things that you can do in life are meditating, focusing, and imagining the life beyond your fondest dreams. You can do this with a vision board and use it as an external visual focus. You can also utilize a longer visualization process. However, this internal visualization requires certain brain parts to be working optimally. Some of these brain parts, or "hardware," change shape and function with chronic stress and chronic pain, which can make it difficult, if not impossible, for some people to visualize or focus on anything for a significant period of time. When focusing is not possible, you want to do more of the active mindfulness exercises, such as breathing exercises, bilateral stimulation, and mindful movement.

Bilateral stimulation exercises stimulate the hemispheres of the brain to balance circulation and activity. There is music that offers this stimulation, including music from hemi-sync.com and Jeffrey Thompson (www.scientificsounds.com). Dr. Thompson founded and directs the Center for Neuroacoustic Research in California. There is a ton of science behind the instrumental music that he has created. It's a mix of various nature sounds as well as instruments. You can find all sorts of "binaural" music online, but not all of it has research backing its effectiveness. Nevertheless, bilateral stimulation is stimulating the brain with different sounds in each speaker, so using headphones is necessary for this to be most effective.

I'm also going to teach you something called tapping or EFT, which stands for Emotional Freedom Techniques. There is an app called the

"Tapping Solution" that you can download, which talks you through the process. I'm going to teach you how to create your own scripts. (See page 102 for more information about tapping.)

EFT can include a bilateral stimulation process when simultaneously tapping on both sides of the body, which is similar to Eye-Movement Desensitization and Reprocessing (EMDR). EMDR, as a therapeutic approach, can be very intense for anyone with chronic pain. I'm not necessarily recommending EMDR, but if you have found it helpful in the past with a licensed professional therapist, you will definitely find EFT useful.

In summary, if meditations or visualization or mindfulness exercises don't feel accessible to you yet, particularly when you're in a pain flare, just go straight to bilateral stimulation. It's going to help the hemispheres of your brain communicate and shift your ANS within minutes.

EXERCISE: DEFINE HEALING

Now I want you to write what healing looks like to you. When's the last time you thought about that? Pain and fear hijack the brain, and when that happens, you tend to only think about what that looks like. Is that true for you? Fear and worry guide you to use your imagination to conjure a world where it never gets better. Therefore, I want you, right now, to intentionally think about what healing looks like to you. Focus on all five senses. Fast forward to the dream. Fast forward to when your body has healed and when life has healed and when you're living the life you love and loving the life you live. Write down your answers to these questions:

- What are you seeing?
- What are you hearing?
- What are you smelling?
- What are you tasting?
- What are you feeling physically?
- Where are you?
- Who's with you? Are you alone?
- What are you doing?

Dedicate 5 to 10 minutes of intentional time every day to thinking about this. You have to remind your subconscious, your brain, your body, and your spirit about what you want on a daily basis. This takes practice.

Remember the concept of sports psychology: If you think about when you missed the basket, guess what? You're most likely going to miss the next basket, right? Sports psychology is all over these different concepts that I'm going to teach you. Pain and fear hijack the brain, so you need to hijack it back! Look at what you wrote for your vision, and offer yourself the opportunity to create your vision board. A vision board is where you print/draw/color images and words that help you remember what healing looks like to you.

Increasing Awareness of the Mind-Body Connection

Now we're going to start moving into increasing your awareness of the mind-body connection. Begin by creating a short list—maybe five things—of what brings you pleasure and joy. Here are some examples:

- Puppies
- Hikes in the woods
- Hugs

- Cup of warm tea
- A good brunch (I love brunch with friends!)

 EXERCISE

Alright, your turn! List five things that bring you pleasure and joy. If you can only think of a few right now, that's okay. That is normal for a brain that's been stuck in pain for a while.

Now, I want you to draw an outline of a body.

Mine usually looks kind of like a gingerbread man cookie—that's okay! You don't have to be a professional artist for this exercise. Draw an outline of a body and, as you tune into what brings you pleasure and joy, recognize and draw the sensations that happen in your body. Where do you feel the sensation? What does pleasure and joy physically feel like? Maybe you draw something like this:

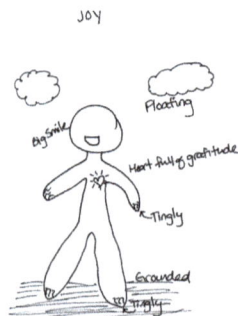

As you draw your experience of joy, you're focusing on how it's experienced physically. For me, I feel a really big smile when I imagine looking at the things that bring me pleasure and joy. I feel lighter so I draw a little bit of clouds around me, and I'm also feeling grounded when I have that warm tea or when I'm walking in the woods. As you see, I drew solid ground beneath my feet. I sometimes feel some tingling in my fingers and my toes when my heart feels happy, so you'll see that I drew some squiggly lines to represent those feelings. What does your drawing show?

Now, I want you to draw another outline of the body. This time, tune into your experience of pain. Draw what happens when you're thinking about the pain.

Pain

For me, my mind gets busy, my stomach tightens, and sometimes I feel prickly in the lower pelvis when I think about pain. I also feel a lot of pressure. Many of us can put pressure on ourselves to figure it out, pressure to push through it, pressure to do X, Y, or Z. Is that true for you? Draw the sensations you are aware of when you tune into your experience of pain.

> Depending on how it ended up in your notebook, you may be able to look at these pictures side-by-side and notice how the physical sensations change depending on what you're thinking about.

These body maps are truly the essence of the mind-body connection. You can't physically feel something without thinking about things, imagining things, remembering things, and vice versa. You can't think about something and remember something without there being a physical response or reaction. There is no separation between the mind and the body, which is why it is sometimes referred to as the "mindbody."

I want you to learn how to utilize your body in terms of breathwork and posture, nutrition and supplements, exercise and relaxation. As you calm your system, you're able to utilize the power of your mind and brain to shift your physical response.

Ultimately, we're either in balance or we're out of balance. You do not want to think of your experience in terms of good or bad. **The body is only your messenger.** The body is giving you feedback. The body is letting you know what you're focusing on by reacting to your thoughts and beliefs. It also lets you know what you're *not* focusing on. This means it's common for many people to be living in a stress response for a prolonged period of time without realizing it or addressing it. Maybe you don't know how to address your stress, so you try to bury it from your consciousness. Maybe you've ignored that Irritable Bowel Syndrome (IBS) for years. Maybe you've gotten into a habit of holding your bowels and bladder for longer than five hours at a time because you didn't want to go to the bathroom at work or you weren't able to get a break from work. Maybe you've learned to work through the smaller discomforts and push through the pain because you observed your caretakers doing that when you were growing up.

Many different things build up cumulatively within the system physically, mentally, spiritually, and emotionally. If you can start to tune into this mind-body connection and tune into the message that your body is trying to tell, you can respond before your body starts to yell.

If you ignore your body's whispers, it will start to yell.

Why do you ignore your body's messages? You're more likely to respond when you feel equipped and resourceful to help your systems manage and process the stress or situation. When you respond and nurture your body, it is going to return to that place of balance and homeostasis, because that's any living creature's main goal: health, vitality, and survival.

Don't Get Lost in the Weeds—Keep it Simple

When you're in fight-or-flight mode, healing slows down. When you're in a calm, restorative state, healing speeds up. The ultimate goal—the top of the pyramid process—is to get to that place where you're calming your nervous system, helping your brain have full function and full communication, imagining the life you love, and dreaming of a life beyond your fondest dreams. Consequently, your body does what you want it to do and what it knows how to do: heal and thrive.

There can be so many different diagnoses and many different things that you can be doing to heal. You want to try to keep it as simple as possible. That becomes possible when you pay attention to your body with an understanding of what's happening and how to respond. Here you see the goal of pain education.

Chapter 3

Pain Education

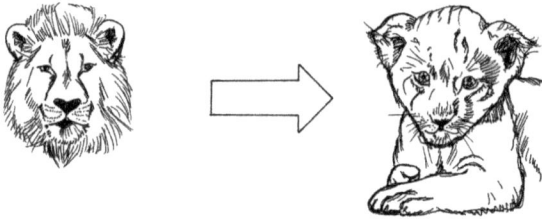

Metaphorically, pain education helps change your understanding and perception of pain from a scary lion to a baby lion. Pain is like a scary lion when you don't understand what's going on in your body, when doctors tell you that it's all in your head, when doctors tell you that they don't know what to do and that it's never going to get better, when you read blogs and read stuff online,* and when you don't know anyone who is experiencing what you're going through.

When pain is a baby lion, there are still things happening in the body. Do baby lions still have sharp teeth and sharp claws? Yes! Is it more manageable than the daddy lion? YES! When you can see a baby lion, you're not scared of it, but you still need to deal with it. When your brain is perceiving a really scary daddy lion, it has a stronger reaction. A stronger reaction in the brain and nervous system is going to lead to increased muscle tension, increased nerve sensitivity, and increased in-flammatory response. **The ANS becomes out of balance when you're scared.** You want to change your brain's perception of pain to seeing it as a baby lion.

---

*Remember most people who write things online are the ones who haven't gotten the resources they need and haven't gotten better. You don't hear enough of the healing stories. Trust me, the healing stories are out there. Over the past 20 years, I have seen hundreds of people heal from CPP, and I share some of their stories in this book.

Research demonstrates that pain education leads to fewer pain flares, less frequency of flares, and decreased intensity of flares. Much of this research is from Lorimer Moseley and David Butler from the Neuro-Orthopaedic Institute of Australia. (I list some of their books in Appendix E.)

Pain education also decreases pain intensity and the habit of catastrophizing. Catastrophizing is when the brain makes a mountain out of a molehill. Unfortunately, it does this automatically without your conscious consent, and it's often due to your brain's hardware changes. Your brain can get stuck in that ruminative cycle. I call it "getting stuck in the traffic circle." You can see this happen on functional MRI scans. (How amazing is that?!) The negative thought or the fear-based thought spins around and around. Every time it goes around, it can feel (and appear) more intense (bigger and brighter on the scan). As you practice the bilateral stimulation and as you understand how pain is processed in the brain, you're going to decrease that catastrophizing, and you will increase your sense of resourcefulness. When you know how to nurture your body, you will feel empowered to take action.

What Is Pain?

Pain used to be thought of as a signal that comes in and then a signal that goes out. It's a lot more complicated than that. Pain is, in fact, "a complex multidimensional event that cannot be reduced to a nociceptive sensation (sensory-discriminative dimension)."* Pain is an *experiential response* by the brain. The signals go up the spine to the brain and, depending on numerous variables, the brain makes a decision and adjusts the dials as to what you are consciously aware of, and how loud that awareness becomes.

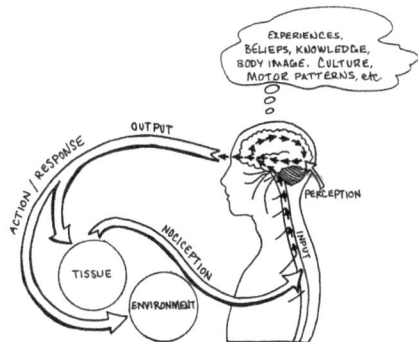

*Janig W. Autonomic reactions in pain. *Pain*. 2012 Apr;153(4):733–735.

Variables that influence your brain's response include, but are not limited to, your:

- Brain's hardware changes
- Brain's circulation and oxygenation
- Past experiences
- Generational trauma
- Beliefs about the body, particularly that part of the body
- Importance of that part of the body
- Cultural experiences
- Current emotional status
- Current overall health status
- Brain's reserve (more on this later)
- And much more!

Your experience is like a soup of all of these variables, and the ingredients can change in a moment's notice—the amount of each ingredient, the size, and the intensity. All of these variables and more get thrown into consideration when the brain is choosing how it wants to respond. **Pain is an output of the brain based on its perception.** You could have major tissue damage and not feel it if your brain is focused on something else or chooses that something else is a higher priority to survival. You want to change the ingredients in the soup of your mind in order for your life to taste better and for physical healing to occur.

Acute versus Chronic Pain

Acute pain serves as a warning or alarm system. Acute pain relates to a sensation in the body that is a result of injury, such as a cut, a broken bone, or a heart attack. Acute pain sends a signal, also called nociception, through the nervous system to the brain, telling the brain something is wrong and needs attention. This process is practically instantaneous, which helps one seek help and medical care as quickly as possible. The electrical component of the nervous system aids in this fast transaction. The signals from the injured area travel through the nervous system to the brain and trigger the alarms. When these signals are sent up the spine and into the brain, the "fight, flight, or freeze" response kicks in.

This is the sympathetic phase of the nervous system. The opposite is the parasympathetic phase, which is the calm restorative phase of the body's nervous system.

The sympathetic phase is an evolutionary protective response. When the "fight, flight, or freeze" response happens, physiological changes take place, including muscle tension, increased heart rate, shallow breathing, and other autonomic nervous system responses, such as dry mouth, slower immune response, and inhibited digestion. During this response, the brain is also checking in with other parts of the body, in what researchers call the "neural pain matrix" or "neuro-matrix." When these signals reach the brain, they are evaluated by different parts of the brain, including the motor cortex and the sensory cortex.

The signal also travels to other parts of the brain where thoughts, memories, and knowledge of our bodies are stored. As seen in functional MRI images, the neuro-matrix can be observed as different parts of the brain light up when these signals and triggers are "set off" in the body or surrounding environment. The brain is looking at the neuro-matrix, which is the accumulation of past experiences (those consciously remembered and those not remembered, from birth to the present moment), beliefs, thoughts focused on throughout the day, the emotional state, and the overall understanding of the situation. This process happens in microseconds, without one's conscious control. This process can decrease or increase one's experience of pain, depending on the perceived "danger" level of those signals.

For example, if someone trips on a curb and sprains their ankle, will it hurt? Most likely, it will hurt. However, if someone trips on a curb and sprains an ankle, but there is a big bus coming toward them, are they going to feel their ankle? They most likely will not feel their sprained ankle until they are safely out of the way of the bus. This phenomenon is the neuro-matrix at work. The brain's perception changes based on what is going on around or within the person. It perceives what is going on in the environment and determines what is more "dangerous" in the present moment.

However, the brain's perception is not always accurate and not always in one's conscious control. An example of this is a visual illusion, such as a mirage of water on a street on a hot, dry day. When most people see this mirage, they know there really is not a pool of water in the middle of the street, but that it is an optical illusion. Growing up, they have learned what a mirage is, and they know that what their eyes see is not truly accurate.

This happens a lot in sports. For example, you see athletes play in the Super Bowl with a broken ankle or try to finish a basketball game even though they've got a compound fracture. There are many examples of people having major tissue damage with no pain, and then you see examples of people having major pain without any tissue damage.

Have you ever experienced phantom pain? There is a famous story about a construction worker who fell on a large nail that pierced through his boot and caused excruciating pain. When he arrived at the hospital and the medical staff removed the boot, everyone was shocked to discover that the nail had gone between his toes and had never pierced his skin. How does this happen? Watch this quick video, and you may be surprised by what you learn.

This process may be described through this equation:

$$\frac{\text{nociception (chemical signals sent through the nervous system)} + \text{perceived threat/danger level}}{\text{level of reaction/response within the nervous system.}}$$

In other words, the amount of danger signals that are sent up into the brain, plus the level of threat that is perceived in the brain, equals the amount of pain experienced. One's response is based on the main question, "How dangerous is the trigger?" In the context of chronic pelvic pain, particularly for a woman who has not received a comprehensive diagnosis, many questions may arise in her mind. These questions may include: "Why can't the doctors find what's wrong with me?" or "What if it's cancer that they can't see?" or "Will this pain last forever?" Depending on the person's conscious awareness or response to these questions, the brain either perceives safety or danger. The more the brain perceives danger, the more pain is experienced.

When discussing chronic pain, it is important to note that chronic pain is not prolonged acute pain. Once an injury is treated, the acute pain dissipates. Chronic pain, on the other hand, is very different. Chronic pain serves no basic survival function. Chronic pain is the result of the nervous system being in overdrive, constantly sending neurological signals to the brain, telling it there is danger when there is often no specific trigger or catalyst. Chronic pain is the result of our brain interpreting signals through our nervous system long after the actual tissue damage has healed.

Triggers in the nervous system can include one or all of the following: functional systems (bladder, bowel, or uterus/prostate) and structural systems (muscles and ligaments in spasm, nerves firing, tingling, burning, itching of surface tissues), all of which add up in our memories, emotions, and thoughts. When the trigger is a memory, emotion, or thought (conscious or unconscious), it lights up the neuro-matrix connected to our sensory cortex. This phenomenon is similar to "phantom limb syndrome" where the individual experiences pain in a part of the body that is no longer there.

Some doctors may be right in stating that the pain is "all in her head" because all nociception is processed in the brain. However, these doctors are wrong when they claim the people are not "really" suffering from pain. The result is many women silently suffer from chronic pain that interrupts their daily lives and ability to function at work and at home. Thus, chronic pain is the perfect example of the mind-body connection because not only are physical triggers causing pain, but also the reaction or response of the neuro-matrix can cause and even increase the physical and emotional reaction to those systemic triggers.

Brain Maps

The main organ that's involved in pain perception is the brain. This is why healing the brain and retraining the brain are so important. We, being healthcare providers, want you to get the most out of your treatments. Pain changes your brain and changes how your brain perceives the world around you and within you. Pain changes the hardware of your brain, and much more.

Physical and functional changes within the brain stem, spinal cord, neural myelin (the protective coating around nerves), vagus nerve, and functional changes are observed throughout the entire ANS system.

An example of this occurs when a signal has been sent up the spine repeatedly over the course of 10 days. The spine will start to send that signal on its own, regardless of any of the incoming information from the peripheral nerves. That becomes problematic, as you can imagine. Here you have yet another reason to heal the brain and the nervous system.

Unfortunately, you also see changes in the brain and body with medication. For example, opiates and benzodiazepines and various other medications can try to close the doors in an effort to decrease the amount of signals going up to the brain. However, the brain and the body are brilliant at adapting. In response to this blockage, the body creates more doorways! Consequently, when you stop using that medication, pain and anxiety spike because now you have more doors. This process adds to the windup of the nervous system. As your nervous system winds up and becomes more sensitive, your brain maps change.

Your brain can react to something whether it's happening now, yesterday, 40 years ago, or even if it never happened at all. Your brain and nervous system react to what is both real and imagined. For example, you can wake up from a dream and be sweaty and panting with your heart pounding. Another example is when you remember something happy or sad and your physical body reacts to it. Your brain does not know the difference between real and imagined. You need to help your brain heal the hardware and update its software. When a signal is sent up your spine, you only want your brain responding to what is happening right now rather than responding to the cumulative history of all the times that it received a similar signal.

When it comes to brain maps, it's not only your experiences that your brain keeps track of. Your mirror neurons activate and cause your brain to light up in the same way when you observe someone or hear their story. You physically react to watching a movie or someone's grimace. All of this creates an experience in your brain's memory files. Brain maps are an important component to understand when discussing chronic pain and ANS regulation.

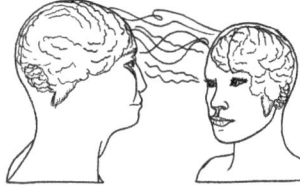

Amit Sood, MD, created a short video to explain the brain's reaction to real and imagined stimuli that can be found on YouTube, called "A Very Happy Brain." Check it out!

Here are five of my favorite books that discuss how your experiences, both real and observed, are stored in the nervous system:

- *The Body Bears the Burden* by Robert Scaer
- *The Body Keeps the Score* by Bessel van der Kolk
- *The Polyvagal Theory* by Stephen Porges
- *My Grandmother's Hands* by Resmaa Menakem
- *Brainscapes* by Rebecca Schwartzman

These books go into depth as to how and why trauma and stress are stored all over the body—both within your physical cells (particularly muscle cells and connective tissue) as well as nerve cells. Sometimes your body remembers things, but your mind does not. Have you ever experienced this? Has your body ever become anxious and reactive to a certain place, smell, or sound and you didn't know why? By tuning into that mind-body connection, you can start to help process things that you may not realize are there. This concept also applies to generational trauma, which is the genetic imprint that ancestral trauma can have in brain mapping. When you put the research from all of these books together, you realize that your body is not only carrying collateral damage that happened during your life, but also during your ancestors' lives.

The body is collateral damage to life.

What causes the brain to click save on these new maps? The brain's job is to keep you safe and help you survive. Therefore, for the brain, it is more important to remember what the dangers are than it is to remember what feels safe and secure. Consequently, you have what is called state-dependent memory and learning (SDLM). This means that when you are in a certain state of being—such as in fight-or-flight mode—the memories and experiences during that state are labeled accordingly, similar to a soundtrack of a movie. When you hear a certain soundtrack, your brain remembers the scene of the movie during which that soundtrack played. Your brain works the same way. When you are in a certain emotional "soundtrack," all the memories you have with that same soundtrack come to the forefront.

The same thing goes for feeling peaceful and relaxed, though these memories are not prioritized as much. Nevertheless, when we're peaceful and relaxed, it's a lot easier to remember all of the memories.*

The emotional state that we're in dictates what information, evidence, memories, and ideas feel most easily accessible. Therefore, when your system has been stuck in fight-or-flight mode, the stress and the trauma that you've experienced are at the top of the "queue" in terms of thoughts and rumination. The solution? More bilateral stimulation. Bilateral stimulation is how you can manually help the brain neutralize the soundtrack and place traumatic memories in the archives. (See page 23.)

Decades of research has been conducted on all of these concepts. **It's never just the body, and it's never just the mind. It's everything**.

All of the exercises you will learn in this book are simple and easy to apply. Sustainable healing requires persistence, repetition, and dedication to practicing these techniques.

---

*A great Pixar movie that talks about these concepts is *Inside Out*, where the creators describe neurobiology to five-year-olds. I recommend watching this movie for a playful demonstration of the SDML concept.

Chronic pelvic and sexual pain is similar to *and* different from chronic pain in other parts of the body.

Chronic pelvic and sexual pain is similar to chronic pain in other areas of the body, and at the same time, it's quite different. CPP is similar to chronic pain in terms of how it's processed in the spine, the brain, and the nervous system. All pain is part of the same nervous system, and it's guided by the same brain, and it all creates a stress response. Chronic pain and CPP change the brain in the same way and require healing in the same way.

However, when you think about brain mapping and the mental representations of the body within the sensory motor cortex, pelvic and sexual pain is very different. The more you use a certain part of your body, the more "real estate" it has in your brain.

The pelvis is at the core of what you do and how you move, and it affects your ability to interact with other people. For example, if you enjoy connecting and interacting with others through athletics, outdoor activities, or exercise, pelvic and sexual pain limits your ability to participate in these activities. The way pelvic and sexual pain affects your everyday life and ability to connect with others, and holds greater real estate in your brain, creates a larger reaction in your nervous system when your brain perceives something is wrong.

The pelvis is also a difficult part of the body to rest and rejuvenate because you're always using it. It's not like a broken ankle that you can rest. The pelvis and genitals can't rest. You need to pee and poop every day, digest food every day, and sit, stand, walk, and move every day. Right? You can't rest the pelvis because you're always using it! That's why it can take longer for these pelvic areas to heal.

The pelvic and sexual regions are also private areas. Too many therapists and healthcare providers tend to shy away from talking about that part of the body, be it anatomy (the parts) or physiology (the function). Often, it's simply because it happens to be in the same part of the body that you have sex in, and no one wants to talk about sex. Also, you learn not to talk about peeing and pooping and periods. It's almost as if most people have an aversion to talking about our most natural functions.*

It often feels very isolating for folks navigating these issues. We've successfully normalized talking about cancer—but not cancer in the genitals. Anyone can feel comfortable talking openly about migraines or chronic pain in the extremities. But more often than not, it can be really hard to talk about pelvic and sexual pain, including any issues with that part of the body, such as GI, bladder, or reproductive functioning. This isolation and silencing adds to the shame and embarrassment that most people feel with dysfunction and pain in that area.

Furthermore, it's a main part of the body where your body holds stress, specifically the GI system. All of this adds to the brain's mapping and reactivity to signals from that part of the body.

The more important the part of the body is to you, the louder the response.

What's the good news? You're going to be able to utilize all of the techniques in this book for all of the above.

> **When you have the courage to see life for what it is now and see a purpose in it, you will know what you need to change and how to go about doing it.**

---

*People are always surprised at the ease with which I talk about this stuff. I have to remind my friends and family and clients it's all I talk about every day with all of my clients! Therapists and physicians alike will say that pelvic and sexual pain are "out of their scope." I'm not sure when the pelvic and genital region was separated from the rest of the body, but we need to change this!

✏️▶ EXERCISE: IT'S ALL CONNECTED: CPP ANATOMY 101

What parts of the body do you believe are currently involved in your experience? Check all that apply.

- ☐ Genitals
- ☐ Bladder
- ☐ Upper GI
- ☐ Lower GI
- ☐ Reproductive organs
- ☐ Pelvic floor muscles
- ☐ Pelvic nerves
- ☐ Migraines
- ☐ Back pain
- ☐ Pain all over

If you have CPP, you likely checked most of those boxes. The main organs in the pelvic region, which include reproductive organs, the bladder, and the gastrointestinal (GI) system, are all common "triggers" of CPP. Other triggers include stress, the brain, and systemic inflammation, which are highly affected by the GI system. The muscles, nerves, and connective tissue (fascia) are the parts of the body that both react to those triggers, and they become a trigger when overworked. There is something called "cross-talk," which refers to the anatomy of nerves firing in both directions, stimulating and communicating with the "neighbors" in the environment. An example of cross-talk is when females have a menstrual cycle that engages a change in GI function. Another example of cross-talk is when the GI system is constipated and this creates muscle spasms throughout the abdomen. Consequently, with CPP, you arrive at "the chicken or the egg" question: Which came first?

By the time you're experiencing the pain regularly, they're all involved. **That is why you want to simultaneously work from the "bottom up" and the "top down."** The "bottom up" means addressing the pelvic floor muscles, the nerves, and the organ systems. The "top down" means addressing the brain, stress, and mental, emotional, and spiritual health.

Treatments for the "bottom up" include, but are not limited to, pelvic floor physical therapy, massage, nerve injections, breath work, acupuncture, yoga, Qi Gong, light therapy, GI healing, and sexual and reproductive health. Pelvic floor physical therapists focus on relaxing muscles in and around the pelvis, as well as provide whole-body evaluations to optimize anatomical balance, structural support, flexibility, and posture. Yoga and Qi Gong also support the improvement of physical balance, as well as mental, emotional, and spiritual homeostasis. Light therapy and nerve injections can provide support in the speeding of nerve regeneration and healing as well as calming down the inflammation around the nerves. Of course, evaluating and addressing all issues of structure and function related to the main organs of the pelvis is always an integral part of the process.

Treatments for the "top down" include, but are not limited to, pain education, behavioral health, nutritional and health coaching, spiritual practices, and meditation. Specific interventions that I have found most helpful are included in this book, all of which are supported by the most recent evidence-based literature available.

You want to heal the habitual patterns that can develop in the spinal cord, the vagus nerve, and the brain that start within 10 to 14 days of experiencing pain. The habit of pain needs to be reprogrammed. The bridge between both ends of the body is the brain-gut connection via the vagus nerve and blood circulation. You need your gut to calm down if you want your bladder to heal, as well as if you want your pelvic floor muscles to relax.

You also need to heal your gut because it is a major component of healing your brain. Once you heal your gut and your brain, you can retrain your brain more efficiently, effectively, and sustainably. Once your brain is able to be reprogrammed, you are going to have faster results from the pelvic floor physical therapy as well as any nerve blocks, other injections, or any other intervention that you may receive. **It's all connected**. Take a moment to view the "Complete Anatomy Review" video tutorial and the images below to help you visually connect the dots of your experience. 🌳

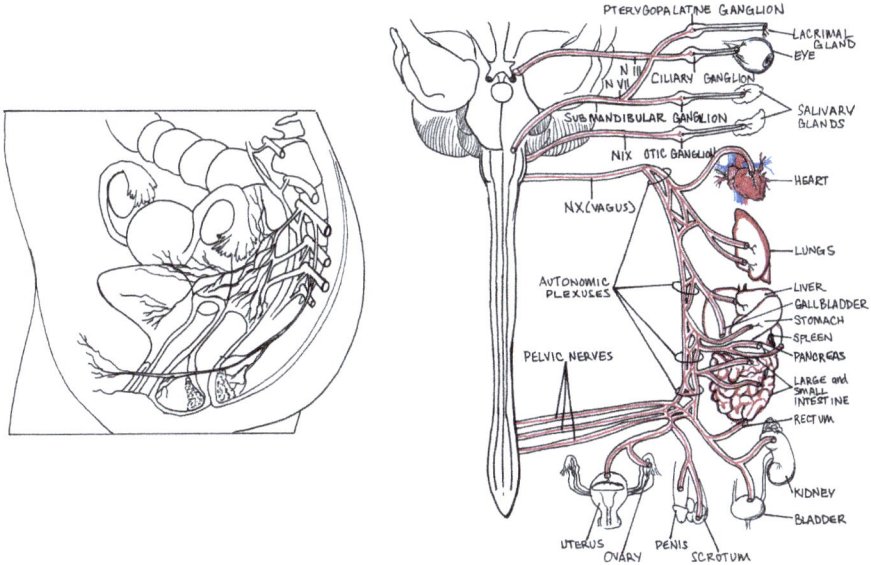

The Vagus Nerve

The vagus nerve is one of the main nerves that is in charge of the entire autonomic nervous system (ANS). **It's also the only nerve that bypasses the spinal cord**. Sometimes you have to use one part of the body to help inform, heal, and update another part of the body.

The vagus nerve travels from the brain all the way down to the pelvic floor, which is why when we're stressed and anxious, the pelvic floor—those layers of muscles in the pelvis—is the first thing that gets tight and tense for most people. Think about it: If I run into a mountain lion, I want my body to go into fight-or-flight mode and "close the tubes" of my pelvis. That's not when it's time to reproduce or poop. Therefore, I want my pelvic floor to do that so I can focus on whatever I need to focus on.

The problem is mountain lions aren't a problem for most people, right? What's the problem? Stress and pain, both internal and external. The pelvic floor always gets engaged when the vagus nerve gets activated, aka when we're in that fight-or-flight mode. Since the vagus nerve physically goes right past the throat, and humming creates a vibration in the back of the throat, this stimulates the vagus nerve and helps calm down the ANS. Rather than just trying to calm the ANS with the mind, we're doing it physically with various exercises, such as the Bumble Bee exercise you practiced earlier. (See page 29.)

The newest science for trauma response, stress response, and chronic pain demonstrate that they are all processed in the same way in the brain, ANS, and vagus nerve. Therefore, utilizing all of the different techniques that I'm going to review is key in reprogramming the painful habits of pain, stress, and trauma.

Common Recommendations for Systemic Healing

There is a strong connection between the brain and the GI system. When one is activated, it activates and agitates the other. If the GI system is upset, it creates angst and anxiety in the mind. When there's anxiety in the mind, the GI system becomes agitated. Therefore, we must work in both directions to calm the system. As we heal the GI system and calm the mind, we significantly decrease systemic inflammation and calm the nervous system sensitivity throughout the entire body, and specifically in the lower pelvic and genital regions. It's all connected!

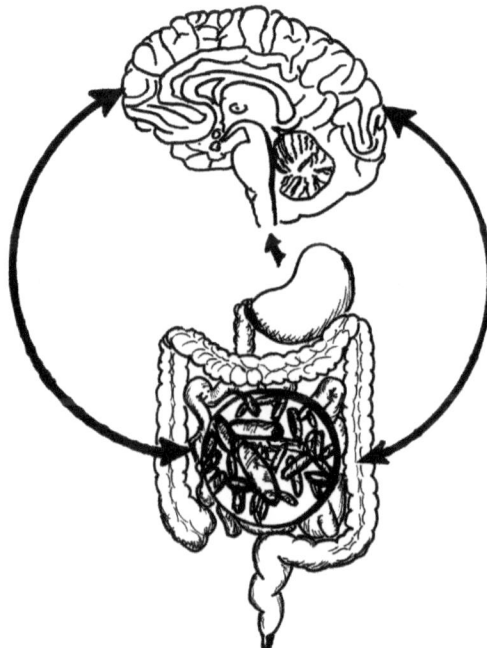

Below you will find supplement and dietary recommendations to heal the GI system. You will also find recommendations for mindfulness and meditation practice, which heal the brain's hardware and improve our ability to click save on new neural habits.

Dietary Recommendations

- 3-week cleanse: Eliminate gluten, dairy, sugar, soy, and corn. If you can only minimize these items, it may take longer for the GI system to heal. It takes 21 days for the GI system to create an entirely new lining and reboot the inflammatory response.

- Substitutions:

  - Scharr brand for gluten-free breads, available at Giant, Wegmans, and Walmart
  - Brown rice or chickpea pasta
  - Multigrain crackers
  - Goat cheese instead of cow cheese: If you must eat cheese, stick with hard, sharp cheeses that have very low amounts of lactose in them
  - Fruit instead of candy, cookies, or sweets
  - Ghee instead of butter

- No matter what, practice this mantra before every meal: ***"Everything I place into my body turns to health and happiness."***

Supplements

- **Reishi mushrooms, turkey tail mushrooms, and lionsmane mushrooms:** (I recommend Host Defense brand.) Reishi and turkey tail balance the immune system and calm inflammation. They come in either capsule or raw form. There is a breadth of research on reishi mushrooms in Chinese Medicine. Lionsmane is fabulous in healing neurological damage and improving neural regeneration in the brain and all over the body. See Paul Stamet's research in the "Fantastik Fungi" documentary available on NetFlix.

- **Vitamin D:** 5000 IU: Boosts immunity

- **DIM:** 200 to 300 milligrams: Calms down the amygdala and decreases excess estrogen in the body, which aids in decreased systemic inflammation and decreased anxiety

- **Zinc:** 25 to 50 milligrams. Boosts immunity, though can cause nausea

- **Magnesium oxide:** 250 to 500 milligrams: Taken at night, helps with muscle and connective tissue relaxation and sleep

- **L-glutamine:** Helps heal the GI system and stimulates cellular regeneration

- **Probiotics** (refrigerated): Helps heal the GI system

- **Iron:** As recommended by your primary care provider

- **Folic acid:** As recommended by primary care provider

- **B1 (thiamine)** or a B-complex vitamin that includes B1: Helps calm the dysautonomia reactions/fight-or-flight response

- **EnteroMend®** (by Health Concerns): Take before or after eating dairy, gluten, sugar, alcohol, soy, and/or corn to decrease inflammatory response

- **Organic food-grade diatomaceous earth:** Take 1 tablespoon in a tall glass of water daily to act as a "binder" and help the body detox faster and more effectively

- **Turmeric:** Anti-inflammatory, useful to add to any meal

Donna Eden's 7-Minute Energy Medicine Routine

Daily Lymphatic Cleanse

- Dry brushing daily before showers (Search YouTube for videos that demonstrate how to do this.)

- Use "T-rex" fingers to gently knead/massage the inside groin and outer thigh, starting at the top and working your way down your thighs to the top of your knee. Then swipe or stroke downward three times as if your trying to dust off the debris. Repeat on the other leg. (To make T-rex fingers, make the peace symbol with your hands, then curl the fingers to look like "T-rex" hands to use your knuckles to massage your body.)

- Follow the lymphatic massage with legs up the wall while lying flat on your back. Roll your shoulders back to open your chest. Place your arms 45 degrees toward the wall. Breathe deeply as you stay in this position for 10 to 15 minutes. Then bring your knees to your chest, roll to your side, and use your hands to help push you up to a seated position. Stay seated for a moment as your blood pressure regulates. Notice how your mind will feel more clear and refreshed.

- Drink a tall glass of water to flush what you just drained out of your system.

Mindfulness, Meditation, Yoga, Qi Gong

- Start with the *Headspace* series available on Netflix. This series offers 20-minute episodes that include 10 minutes of didactic, scientific explanation of meditation and a 10-minute meditation. Each episode offers a different approach to meditation, which can help you realize how accessible this practice can be for your daily life.

- My website and YouTube channel offer a variety of exercises and meditations you will find useful in shifting your mental, emotional, and physical state, returning to homeostasis and optimal well-being. 🌳

- My audio CDs are available on iTunes and Amazon: "Guided Meditations for Mindful Living" and "Guided Meditations for 4-D Healing."

- Iyengar Yoga provides anatomical balance and meditative focus. As you balance the body, you balance the mind and strengthen your sense of self. You can find tutorials online.

- Qi Gong is a gentle, meditative movement that helps balance your energy channels, circulation, and nervous system. You can find tutorials online.

- Jeffrey Thompson instrumental music provides bilateral stimulation to the brain when listened through headphones. It's very effective at calming and healing the brain from trauma, stress, and brain injuries. www.scientificsounds.com

Gut and Bowel Health

We want our stool to come out like soft, raw sausage. Take a look at the Bristol Scale, below. What does your stool look like? You don't want your stool to look like pebbles, but you also don't want it too loose and soft. You want it around a 4 on the Bristol Scale.

BRISTOL STOOL CHART

Type 1 Separate hard lumps, like nuts (hard to pass)

Type 2 Sausage-shaped, lumpy

Type 3 Sausage-shaped, with cracks on the surface

Type 4 Sausage- or snake-like, smooth and soft

Type 5 Soft blobs with clear-cut edges (easy to pass)

Type 6 Fluffy pieces with ragged edges, mushy

Type 7 Watery, no solid pieces (entirely liquid)

Your stool should also feel easy to release—no straining. Straining adds to pelvic floor muscle spasms and inflammation around the pelvic nerves. If you struggle with constipation, bilateral stimulation music, tapping, and breathing exercises can help both before and after a bowel movement. I also recommend a "squatty potty" footstool (available at www.squattypotty.com) that lifts your knees above your hips, as shown below. You can also use any plastic footstool available at a department or big-box store.

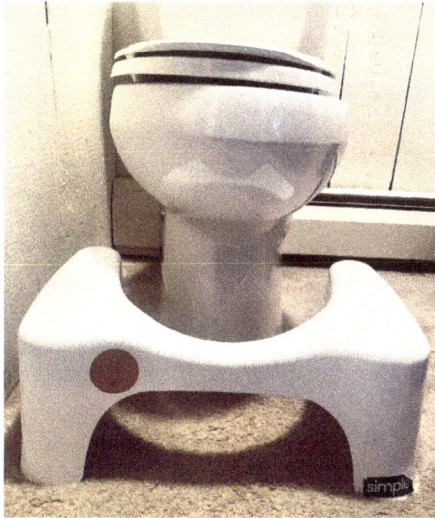

Chapter 4

The Power of Posture and Movement

Posture is more than trying to look proper or influence how others perceive us, like I was taught growing up. Posture affects your emotional and physical functioning. We're going to start with Amy Cuddy's research, which she explores in her book *Presence*.*

Cuddy's research demonstrates that holding an open posture decreases cortisol and increases testosterone. Cortisol is the stress hormone that creates inflammation all over the body, most commonly in the GI system and areas of past trauma or injury. When you're in fight-or-flight mode and in pain, your brain creates more cortisol. Testosterone is the hormone that helps you feel confident, courageous, and energized. Therefore, poor posture increases inflammation and decreases your energy levels.

Poor posture also affects the functioning of your ANS and vagus nerve, as well as increases tension in the low back and pelvic floor. Take a look at these images:

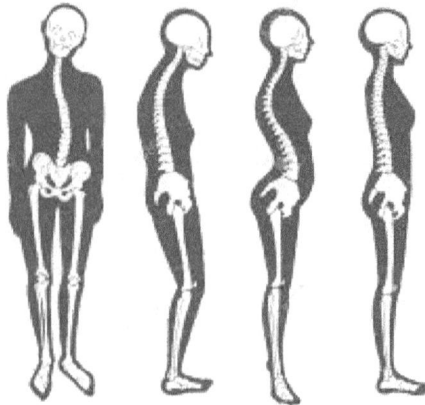

*As with Amy Cuddy's Ted Talk and many other research, there are naysayers and folks who challenge the science. I want you to do the same with me! Challenge some of the information that I share with you. I *also* want you to challenge the information

When you open the front of your spine and uplift your chest, you engage the primary muscles that are meant for supporting your torso on your pelvis. This allows your pelvic floor to relax. Alternatively, when you are curled up, and have a closed posture, that engages your pelvic floor to be the main supporting structure. When you're feeling scared or anxious, you curl up and your pelvic floor engages. When you're standing up and feeling courageous, your back muscles and leg muscles engage. Curling up also puts pressure physically on your vagus nerve, which is the main nerve in charge of the ANS. Therefore, poor posture increases your blood pressure and heart rate, and it limits the depth of your breath because there is less room for your diaphragm to move and less room for your lungs to expand.

Therein lies the irony. When you're scared, your initial reaction is to want to close up. You want to protect your core. You may have your hands, arms, and fists in front of you so you're ready to fight, your head is looking straight ahead, and your tongue is usually in the back of your mouth, which allows you to breathe faster. Meanwhile, if you want to relax the system, you need to do the opposite. This is where the benefits of posture exercises come in.

TRY THIS NOW

Alternate between a closed posture and an open posture. Notice the difference in your breathing.

Let's practice Amy Cuddy's Power Pose. First, in your notebook or on the Activity Record Form (see page 285 in Appendix C), write down your current subjective units of distress (SUDs) level, -10 (worst) to +10 (best). Your pre- and post-SUDs level can be a great way to keep track of which exercise feels more effective for you. Next, create an open posture by placing your hands on your hips. You can also create an

that you read on blogs and hear on podcasts and from your providers. This is how you become your own advocate and engage in your own healing process. It's important to challenge any information that's given.

open posture by placing your arms in the shape of a "V" or any way that helps open the front of the chest. Now, hold that Power Pose for a full two minutes (120 seconds). How do you feel now? Is there a difference in your SUDs level?

Amy Cuddy's science is based on holding poses for two minutes. It is pretty remarkable how much your body's chemistry can shift so quickly.

Something important to note about Power Poses is that even folks born blind, who have never seen anybody else's body language, hold an open posture when they're feeling proud and confident. For example, in paralympic games, congenitally blind athletes hold their hands up in the V pose when they win. Therefore, it is built into your brain mapping to hold a Power Pose when you're feeling excited, proud, and confident. Amy Cuddy is one of many researchers who have demonstrated that the mind can change the body, and the body can also change the mind.

Now I'm going to teach you something called **Reflexercise,** created by Scott Musgrave 🌳. Write down your current SUDs level. You already uplifted the self a little bit through the Power Pose, but this exercise works specifically to calm the nervous system. Reflexercise is simply holding the opposite posture from what the body wants to do when it's in fight-or-flight mode. I learned Reflexercise about 15 years ago when I worked with Robert Echenberg, MD, who was one of the initial pelvic pain specialists in the country. What we would do is test the sensitivity levels of various trigger points on patients before and after holding this posture. They would rate the sensitivity of the point, then perform the postural exercise, then rate their sensitivity again. Every time, without fail, their sensitivity level decreased. It was quite remarkable! Now you're going to experience it. Follow these steps:

1. Curl your toes like you're picking up a pencil.

2. Open your arms and open your palms.

3. Roll your shoulders back. (I remember my yoga teacher would always say open the windows in the front of your armpits.)

4. Turn your head to either side, just as long as it's not looking straight ahead.

5. Close your eyes if you feel safe to do so, otherwise, look down at the floor.

6. Place your tongue against the back of your front teeth or bite your tongue in between your front teeth. As you breathe, you're going to sound a little bit like a snake.

7. Hold all of this while you take three breaths—slow, soft, steady inhalations and exhalations.

8. Keep holding that posture while you intentionally think about someone who's easy to feel love for and take three more breaths.

Now notice how your nervous system feels and record your SUDs level. Both Power Poses and Reflexercise are very effective in how they engage the vagus nerve to calm down the ANS.

Why does Reflexercise work? This posture is doing the opposite of what the body wants to do when we're in fight-or-flight mode. Therefore, when you are experiencing a pain flare, anxiety attack, or even a muscle spasm, you can practice Reflexercise and create a significant shift in your ANS.

> For CPP, Reflexercise can be very helpful after a bowel movement. If you manage pelvic floor spasms or nerve pain after voiding, calming the nervous system directly afterward can be really helpful for two reasons: (1) it calms the nervous system, and (2) it calms the fear response. It's all the same nervous system. Remember, fear, pain, and trauma can hijack the brain so you want to hijack it back. Holding these postures is a way that you can do that.

These are effective postural exercises you can do no matter where you are, and no one really is going to notice that you're doing anything special.

Movements Based in Energy Psychology

I'm now going to teach you a few body movements that are easy to utilize on a regular basis. Donna Eden,* a leader in the Energy Psychology world, has many phenomenal books explaining energy psychology, and the ins and outs of why these movements are effective in bringing the body back into homeostasis. Her energy movements help reset the electromagnetic energy within and around the body. The National Institutes of Health (NIH) calls it the "biofield." (See my list of Energy Psychology Research and Resources on page 298 in Appendix E.)

EXERCISE: GET MOVING

I'm going to share some of my favorite Energy Psychology movements with you. The first is called an **Energetic Shower,** which you can also view on my website). This is useful for when you want to release the residue of a tense conversation or after you've watched the news and now you feel some negativity sticking around you.

Breathe in and hold your hands into fists in front of you as if you're gripping the residue, then release the breath and open your palms as you imagine

---

*Donna Eden is married to David Feinstein, MD, who used to head of the department of psychiatry at Johns Hopkins University. He was aware of psychiatric medications' side effects and limitations. When he met Donna and learned how she healed herself from tuberculosis and multiple sclerosis at a young age, he became fascinated with learning more about energy psychology. After learning about meridian tapping (Emotional Freedom Techniques, or EFT), he left his position and has spent the rest of his life studying the science behind Energy Psychology.

throwing it away. (Maybe you want to imagine throwing it into a fire and watching it evaporate into nothingness.) Now imagine a pool of light in front of you and inhale as you use your hands to scoop the light. With an exhalation, imagine pouring it over you like a shower. Open your posture and bring an intention into the process, such as "I allow this light to cleanse the sticky residue of fear, criticism, and/ or negativity."

With a slow exhalation and open palms face down, slowly move your hands down in front of you as you imagine showering your whole body with the cleansing, healing light. Repeat two more times. Notice how you feel.*

After this exercise try the **Zip-Up Exercise,** also available at my website. 🌳 For this exercise, imagine zipping yourself up, as if you're zipping up a protective shield around you. Start at the pubic bone and imagine zipping up a zipper all the way up your bottom lip. Then start at the bottom of your spine and imagine you're zipping up a dress. Use your imagination to pull that zipper all the way up to your neck and zip all the way up and around your head to the top lip. I find that this Zip-Up Exercise can help uplift the system.

---

*The research on these exercises is fascinating. You can now measure the electromagnetic frequency that's emitted from the body. You see it go from a chaotic energy field to more balanced energy field. This correlates with a calmer blood pressure, quieter brain waves, and calmer heart rate. More of that science to come later.

Next, place two fingers on your belly button and two fingers between your eyebrows. Gently push in and pull up. This usually that inspires you to take a deep breath, especially if you needed to take one. Notice if your body automatically took that deep breath. That means it's working! Try that again. How did it make you feel? Make a note about these exercises in your notebook.

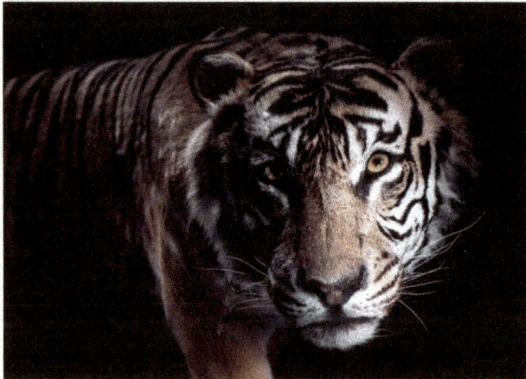

THE TIGER'S STORY

Tara Brach, a leader in the mindfulness world, tells a story in one of her books about a Siberian tiger that lived in an 11-by-11-foot cage for many years. When the tiger was finally rescued and put on a large natural preserve, it stayed pacing in an 11-by-11-foot space. It took months before the staff could coerce the tiger to move outside of that small space.

I share this story to highlight, once again, the importance of dreaming and practicing in your mind what healing looks like. The brain remembers stories more than didactic talking points. I seek to emphasize the importance of dreaming of a better life and dreaming of your greatest self. Let's say you wake up tomorrow and the pain is gone. Then what? Are you ready for that? How would you live your life differently? Would you go back to living the way you were before?

If pain's main message is to slow down and live a more balanced lifestyle, have you received the message and applied it to your new life? If you've been trapped by this chronic pain for months, let alone years, you can get into the habit of not even thinking about healing.

If the mind is the architect and the body is the builder, you need to provide the blueprint of what you want! When you stop giving your body the blueprint of what you want, your body tends to just click "repeat." That's what happened with the tiger. Therefore, plan for how you want to live your life differently once you've healed.

The Brain's Reserve

Have you ever wondered why trauma affects some people more than others? The brain has only so much bandwidth before it runs out of space and the system feels overwhelmed. It's like a car that runs out of gas. See the image on the next page.

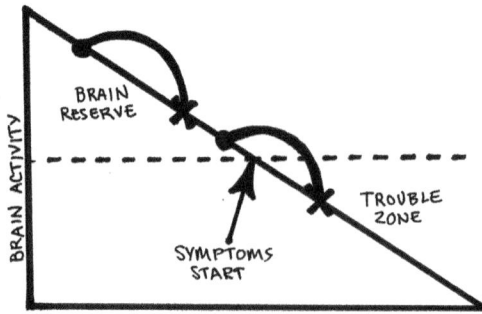

If you start with a full tank of gas and you experience a long "road trip" or traumatic experience, you can endure a lot longer before you run out. However, if you start the long road trip on a half-tank of gas, you're going to run out of energy a lot faster. If you don't take care of yourself by practicing techniques that help your brain clear out the trash (like the "cookies" and the "cache" on your computers), your system will run slower and start to malfunction. Your brain is a complex computer. If too many programs are running at the same time, the computer processing slows down. Likewise, trauma and stress build up in your system. Then, when you experience one more trauma, that takes you below your reserve and then you're in the trouble zone. This is when chronic physical symptoms start to occur.

Keep this in mind when thinking about your own life and your own brain map. Sometimes I'm working with someone and they'll say, "When I look back on my life, I feel like I had a good life. I don't feel like I experienced any trauma." They go on to describe a beautiful childhood with a sense of safety, privilege, and success. *Then* the other stories come out—stories of having to care for ailing parents while getting a divorce and selling their childhood home and navigating a new job during a pandemic. Even if you've had a "picture perfect" life, you can't live in this world without experiencing various levels of stress and trauma. Furthermore, as discussed earlier in Dr. Sood's video, observing trauma or hearing about the pain and suffering of others becomes part of your own brain map.

Especially in the past 10 years, the amount of information that your brain is receiving on a regular basis has grown exponentially. With the internet, social media, and news at your fingertips, your brain's reserve is overwhelmed. You are bombarded by hundreds of notifications daily. Every time a new news article or social media post pops up on your phone, your brain reacts. Your systems are overwhelmed with information, commentary, and the emotional experiences of friends, family members, and even strangers.

Your brain lights up in the same ways as that other person's brain is lighting up, whether they're in front of you or on a screen. If you're in a career field such as law, therapy, or medicine, or your job is to talk to people in crisis on a regular basis, your brain is experiencing everything that they share with you. That's a lot of bandwidth getting taken up by the world around you. You have to think about that.

Brain Hardware Changes

Daniel Amen, MD, is one of the foremost physicians and researchers in neuroscience highlighting the need to look at the brain as an organ when it comes to treating mental illness. Whether it's anxiety, depression, bi-polar disorder, post-traumatic stress disorder (PTSD), or attention deficit disorder (ADD), this abstract concept of mental illness has been attempted to be understood in terms of neurochemicals in the brain. Dr. Amen has spent 30 years looking at brain scan images and the activity levels in the brain.

The images at that site compare a healthy brain that has full, balanced, symmetrical activity with a brain that experienced two strokes. In this example, the strokes create damage and decreased activity in the right hemisphere of the brain. The other images on the right show what happens to the brain with chronic stress, chronic pain, and trauma. Dr. Amen's research, and many other neuroscience research over the past 20 years, demonstrates that similar hardware changes occur with chronic stress, chronic pain, and trauma.

If you want to think differently and feel differently, you must look at healing the organ of the brain.

Within 10 days of experiencing chronic pain and chronic stress, brain hardware changes start to occur. I'm going to highlight a few of the changes here. (For a longer list and description of brain hardware changes, see "The Overlap Between Areas of the Brain Affected by Trauma and the Areas of the Brain Required for Female Sexual Desire" on page 80.) The first, and perhaps the most important, change you see is with the amygdala, which is the part of the brain that is responsible for the activation of your sympathetic nervous system, or fight-or-flight mode. After 10 days of being in this mode, the amygdala's new default mode is "fight-or-flight." Everything in your environment is deemed unsafe until proven otherwise. It's a "guilty until proven innocent" perspective the brain now takes. The amygdala seems to forget how to turn off.*

The amygdala is now on, rather than off, the majority of the time. When that happens, you see changes in the hippocampus. The hippocampus is one of the main memory chips in the brain. The hippocampus is supposed to be the size of a double peanut M&M'S (my favorite candy). Within about 10 days of being in either pain or chronic stress, it changes to look more like a melted M&M'S. It literally starts to flatten out and malfunction. That is when you can expect to have short-term and long-term memory loss, difficulty multi-tasking, and difficulty being able to keep the brain focused on what you're doing or planning to do. You may even learn to blame these things on age, but it's actually the hardware change in your brain.

The pituitary gland also starts to malfunction, which leads to endocrine changes and hormone fluctuations and imbalances. There can be flares with endometriosis, hair growth, ovarian cysts, and fibroids, and women might get their periods at weird times or not at all. Many different things start to happen when the pituitary gland malfunctions.

---

*When you're working with a nervous system that's revved up for a long time, you can't calm it down too abruptly because that's going to feel unfamiliar. You want to gradually calm the nervous system in a way that feels safe and comfortable.

The anterior cingulate cortex (ACC) is a horseshoe-shaped part of the midbrain that is one of the main hardware parts responsible for the communication between the left and right hemispheres of the brain. (Remember what I said earlier about bilateral stimulation and the importance of hemispheric communication?)

The cerebral cortex, which is the gray matter that surrounds the whole brain, is also responsible for hemispheric communication. Chronic pain and stress can cause the cerebral cortex to shrink and lose significant mass, sometimes up to 50 percent! If you think of your cerebral cortex as one of the main highway systems between the left and right hemispheres, that's a lot fewer lanes. Talk about a traffic pileup! When those four major parts of the brain change, it paves the way for it to be harder for the brain to process everyday things.

> The hemispheres of the brain are physically separate from each other for survival reasons. If you have a stroke or a head injury, it doesn't result in complete system shutdown because the separation helps save the other side of the brain. This is why strokes often affect only one side of the brain.

Consequently, you have a shorter fuse. You feel stressed and overwhelmed more easily. Your "computer" runs slower, just like your laptop if you have too many programs running at once, or if you haven't cleaned out the trash, cookies, and cache in a while. If your tech toys malfunction when they don't get cleaned out and turned off every day, how do you think your complex brain reacts when you don't do the same?

You also see changes within the hypothalamus, the thalamus, and the limbic system—all of which navigate the main emotional centers of the brain. In brain scans, researchers discovered a diamond-shaped pattern with chronic trauma, stress, and pain. It makes it look like "the bridge is out" so to speak, between the left and right hemispheres as well as between the posterior and the anterior cortex. This makes it more challenging for the brain to work the way it's created to work.

That is why you move into the bilateral stimulation as your first line of defense. You have to manually plug in your brain through physical stimulation of the left and right sides of the body to help wake up that connection between those two hemispheres. You want the brain to be connected and intertwined so everything can work the way it's supposed to work.

The Overlap Between Areas of the Brain Affected by Trauma and the Areas of the Brain Required for Female Sexual Desire*

1. **Vagus nerve:** Stephen Porges and his Polyvagal Theory have done much to bring attention to the role of the vagus nerve in trauma and trauma release. The vagus nerve plays an important role in the expression and management of emotions. When the mind is triggered into an arousal state, the body is alerted through stored connections, and this information is relayed by the vagus nerve. The vagus nerve is also the connection between the genitals and the brain.

2. **Amygdala:** The amygdala is the brain's alert center. It consists of two almond-sized bundles of neurons that sit on top of the right and left hippocampus. It is primed to be sensitive to fear, danger, and anxiety, regardless of whether the perceived danger is due to a mugging in a dark alley or to an attachment issue. The amygdala communicates with the hypothalamus, cingulate gyrus, brain stem, hippocampus, orbital frontal cortex, and septal nucei, evaluating information from each of these regions regarding the welfare of the person.

3. **Insula:** The insula plays an important role in internal body awareness (interoception), emotion, and consciousness. Other functions include self-awareness, interpersonal experience, cognitive functioning, perception, and motor control.

*Adapted with permission from Keesha Ewers ©2015 Academy for Integrative Medicine

4. **Anterior cingulate gyrus**: Located in the front of the brain, it is a cortical region that often influences cognition. This region is responsible for distinguishing between safe and dangerous, past from present, and relevant from non-relevant. "Talk therapy" cannot access this part of the brain. This is where trauma-release modalities such as Brainspotting, EMDR, or hypnotherapy are therapeutic.

5. **Brain stem:** The brain stem controls the basic functions of heart rate, breathing, and blood pressure, as well as sleeping and arousal and assimilation of nutrition and elimination. We must make sure we "stabilize the fort" and regulate these core functions before doing any trauma release. None of these functions are responsive to talk therapy. We cannot argue our way out of hyper-arousal, talk ourselves into better digestion, or tell ourselves to go to sleep.

6. **Limbic system:** Known as the emotional system of the brain, the limbic regions process information from so many sources that are coming and going in so many directions that it can influence much of our thinking and action. The structures of the limbic system are responsible for processing emotions, motivation, survival states, and feelings about relationships. Early attachment experiences that lead to either feelings of security or feelings of anxiety in the developing child are processed here.

7. **Hippocampus:** The hippocampus is responsible for the ability to store and retrieve memories. Along with other limbic structures, the hippocampus also plays a role in a person's ability to overcome fear responses.

8. **Hypothalamus:** The hypothalamus links the endocrine system and the brain via the **pituitary gland**. It receives alerts from the **amygdala** when there is a perceived or real threat of danger. It then activates the fight-or-flight responses via the brain stem and spinal cord. It also sends messages to the pituitary, which in turn stimulates the adrenal glands to release stress and sex hormones.

9. **Orbital frontal cortex (OFC):** OFC abnormalities or reduction in volume have been reported in mood disorders, anxiety disorders, personality disorders, drug addiction, schizophrenia, and PTSD.

10. **Thalamus:** When we undergo a traumatic event our **thalamus**, which weaves temporal and sensory information into a story that can clarify who we are, where we are, and what we are doing, disconnects. Additionally, the **prefrontal cortex**, which integrates past, present, and future, and is the home of our working memory, also goes offline. This is the mechanism of flashbacks and getting "stuck" in a rumination loop of negative thoughts.

The Effect of Hardware Changes

Let's review the effects of hardware changes. Circle the ones that apply to you.

- Altered perception
- Diminished executive functioning
- Decreased inhibition (You're more likely to be impulsive and go for that that quick fix. This is why it's easier to develop unhealthy habits and addictions.)
- Disrupted sleep patterns (Once this starts, the domino effect begins on an upregulated and dysfunctional nervous system.*)
- Working memory disruption
- Short- and long-term memory loss
- Mood fluctuation
- Anxiety and depression
- ANS dysregulation

More behavioral results of these brain hardware changes include:

- Anger
- Aggressiveness
- Defensiveness
- Reactive/hypervigilance
- Impulsiveness
- Poor focus/attention

---

* Sleep medications actually prevent your brain from falling into a deep, restorative sleep. While the medication may knock you out, it stops your brain around stage 2 or stage 3 of sleep. For neural and cellular regeneration, you need your brain to drop into stages 4 to 5. The brain exercises I teach you in the book will help guide your brain into deeper relaxation and deeper sleep levels.

- Sleep disturbances and nightmares
- Bossyness/need for control
- Lack of empathy
- Increased anxiety and panic disorders
- Fatigue
- Tantrums in children (and adults)
- Fidgety
- Irritability
- Rapid mood fluctuations
- "Never enough" mindset
- Delays in reaching physical, language, or other developmental milestones

Long-term effects of these hardware changes include:
- Upregulated nervous system, or "central sensitization"
- Chronic pain
- Anxiety/panic disorders
- Autoimmune diseases
- Increased systemic inflammatory response
- Post-traumatic stress disorder

Two books that go into these manifestations and provide hope for healing include *Solving the Autoimmune Puzzle* by Keesha Ewers and *The Fear Cure* by Lissa Rankin, MD. Dr. Rankin shares an abundance of success stories about how when you are able to calm down and heal the autonomic nervous system, diseases (even cancers) and chronic pain are able to heal.

To help us understand the brain's reserve and why chronic stress, trauma, and pain create these changes, Lorimer Moseley and David Butler use a metaphor of a bathtub in their patient handbook, *The Explain Pain Handbook: Protectometer.* Life events, injuries, traumas, and stressors fill up the bathtub. The event that triggers the pain is what overflows the tub, so that's what you blame for the pain. When discussing their pain, some people will say to me, "It just came out of the blue" or "I don't understand; it wasn't even a hard fall." You tend to blame whatever happened when the pain started, rather than understanding the initial build-up within the nervous system.

For example, in whiplash research, scientists explored why some people can walk away from an accident while others end up with chronic pain. When we're looking at brain maps, you have to recognize what else is in the bathtub. Write the answers to these questions in your notebook: What filled up your nervous system? What has been taking up space and bandwidth in your brain? **It's the accumulation of trauma, stress, and pain that creates the habit of chronic pain.**

Metaphorically, once the water overflows (once your system is overwhelmed), the tissue tolerance goes down. Before the sensitization occurs, and before the habit of chronic pain, the nerves need to be stimulated to a certain intensity before they choose to send the signal and be "heard" by the brain. Think about it: if you felt every single sensation, your brain would be overwhelmed. Your brain can only handle so much information at the same time.

For example, I can't be aware of how my pinky toe, my heel, my ankle, my elbow, my shoulder, etc., etc. feel all of the time. A lot of unimportant information is in your sensory awareness, and it's simply not necessary for survival. Over time, when pain or injury start to happen cumulatively in one part of the body, the tissue tolerance goes down, and it takes a lighter and lighter touch to set off the same heightened signal.

The image on the next page is one way to visualize this concept. Keep in mind, as you heal the brain and nervous system, your tissue tolerance is going to go back up. Until you really address everything that's going on in your brain map, as well as heal the nervous system by retraining it to be calm, the tissue tolerance will be lower. Lower tissue tolerance equals a louder response to smaller stimulus.

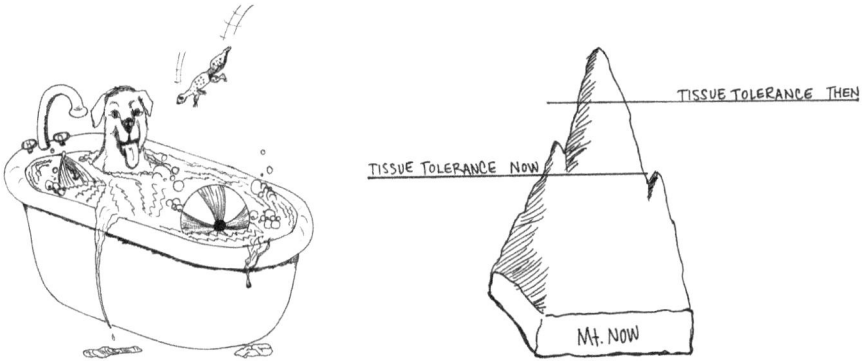

You also see changes in the in the spinal cord. Where the nerve signals go into the spine, there is something called the dorsal root ganglia or the DRG. The DRG in the spinal cord is like the bouncer at the bar: It chooses what signals come in and what signals don't come in. The DRG is really important because it's saying, "OK, all of you signals, you're not really important. She doesn't need to know about all that's going on," or, "Oh! You're an important signal because you've been coming to me all day every day for a while now. I'm going to let you in."

What you see with chronic stimulation—such as if you're a truck driver and sit all day, have painful periods that last seven-plus days, or have an injury that isn't managed—the spinal cord lets more signals in, and it can also start to send the signal on its own. When the DRG starts to receive information on a chronic basis of a certain intensity, the DRG will prioritize that signal and start to send the signal on its own.

Over time, the DRG can actually disappear due to overstimulation. When that happens, there is no longer a bouncer at the bar, and all the signals go in. On one hand, that's bad news. Research demonstrates that once the DRG dies off from overstimulation, it doesn't grow back. On the other hand, the body can reroute itself and create new neural connections, kind of like creating a new central station within the spinal cord. How amazing is that?! However, this takes intentional training, visualization, persistence, repetition, and dedication.

When it comes to pain, accurate perception is vital. When evaluating how Western medicine tends to approach the body in a segmented way, you forget that it's all connected. For example, a GI specialist will only look at the GI system, a gynecologist is only going to look at the reproductive system, and a urologist is only going to look at the bladder and kidneys. The majority of experts forget to look at the nerves and the muscles in the pelvis entirely.

I like to share this parable, especially in the realm of chronic pelvic and sexual pain:

> *Two people are in a boat, and one of them is making a hole in the boat. The other one says, "What are you doing?! You're destroying us!" The first person says, "Oh, don't worry, I'm just making this hole in my part of the boat."*

Growing up, many of us learned to segment the body into parts. Western medicine has a different specialty for every organ and every body part. **You must remember that the whole body is connected, and the whole nervous system is connected**. You need to shift perspective and zoom out to see the broader picture, the whole picture.

Chapter 5

Shifting Perspective

S hifting perspective takes practice. Mindfulness can help. When I began learning about mindfulness and these brain exercises to shift perspective, I learned it from skydiving.

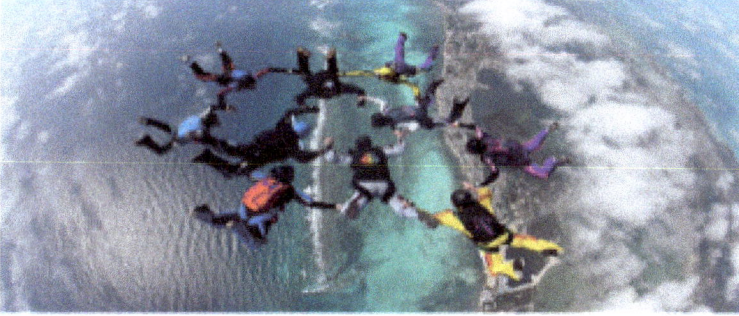

That's me with the red parachute, and that's my dad in the yellow suit. We learned how to skydive together, and it was really quite an amazing journey. The blue roofs below his left knee was the only landing area!

What I love about this memory is remembering when my skydiving instructor handed me the book *The Power of Now* by Eckhart Tolle, saying, "Alex, if you don't learn how to be in the moment, you're going to die in this sport!" Nothing like some good ol' fear-based teaching. With skydiving, you need to be aware of your body position, wind speed, altitude, and other skydivers—similar to defensive driving on the highway. There's a lot to keep track of and a lot on the line if something gets missed.

Being in the sky certainly brings perspective when you get to see the earth from that high up. Not many people get to see earth from the clouds' and birds' perspective.

When I'm in fight-or-flight mode, I remember my skydiving instructor's advice, and I think about what else is going on around me. That's what you want to do when you're in a pain flare. You want to zoom out and ask, "What are all the different factors that could be adding to my pain right now?"

Ideally, through the practice of mindfulness and practicing shifting your perspective, you'll guide your nervous system back to a place of observation. You'll recognize that you are not that sensation, you are not that thought, you are not that emotion. You are the observer. Rumi stated, "I am not this hair. I am not this skin. I am the soul that lives within."

As you shift to the observer perspective, you can explore and discover the meaning that you've placed on things. You can start to move some pieces around the board, such as asking yourself, "What if I change the meaning I've placed on this pain?"

What possibilities come into your awareness as you shift perspective? Saint Francis of Assisi stated, "What you're looking *for* is already where you're looking *from*."

The nervous system travels at 240 miles an hour, so by the time you think about looking for the pain, you've already unintentionally recreated (and sometimes amplified) it, through fear-based memory.

Do you have any perspectives about your pain that you want to shift? As you walked the 4-D Wheel, did you become aware of any new perspectives? As you explore your brain map, you can gain awareness of the variables that go into what either amplifies, or calms down, your brain's perspective on pain.

Zooming out and changing perspective can remind us of the process of nociception and how brains have different reactions based on perspective. Let's explore what could be in your brain map and adding to your brain's perspective of your pain.

✏️➤ EXERCISE: CREATING THE 2-D AND 4-D TIMELINE OF YOUR BRAIN'S MAP

Place your notebook in landscape position so you have enough room. You may even want to do this over two pages. Draw a line to represent the timeline of your life. Mark when you were conceived, leaving room before that to note generational trauma. Mark when you were born, and put a star for where you are currently, leaving space for the future to write your dreams and goals. Now, note any traumatic events or unpleasant events on the bottom of the timeline (i.e. mother's stress during pregnancy, pneumonia as a baby, and broken bones or injuries). Note any pleasant events on the top of the timeline (i.e. winning a sports game, a memorable vacation, graduating high school or college, getting a promotion). Using a long curved line, note long-term events (i.e. alcoholic parents and stressful childhood home, painful periods from teenage years to current time, two years of a pandemic, a divorce process, difficult pregnancy symptoms).

The important part of this is to recognize how many events were overlapping and the emotional stress that added to your brain's experience and *perception* of the physical events that happened. For example, maybe a loved one died of COVID, so there was a lot of grief at the same time when you went through a surgery and needed to be alone in the hospital during recovery. You might not be able to write down everything, but for now, note the events that stand out to you. You can always add to it later. Once complete, you have created the two-dimensional timeline of your life.

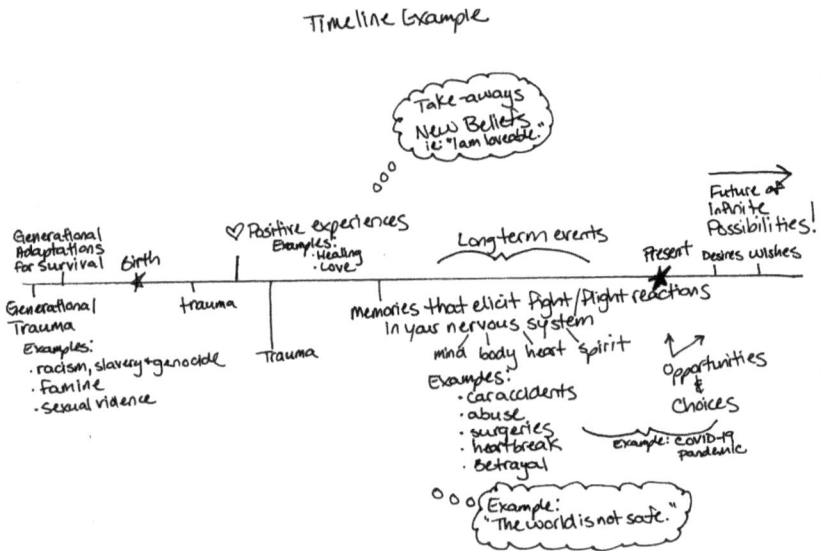

Timeline Example

Take-aways
New Beliefs
ie: "I am loveable."

Generational
Adaptations
for Survival   Birth

♡ Positive experiences
Examples:
· Healing
· Love

Long-term events

Present

Future of
Infinite
Possibilities!
Desires wishes

Generational
Trauma
Examples:
· racism, slavery + genocide
· Famine
· Sexual violence

trauma

Trauma

memories that elicit fight/flight reactions
in your nervous system
mind body heart spirit
Examples:
· car accidents
· abuse
· surgeries
· heartbreak
· betrayal

Opportunities
&
Choices

Example: covid-19
pandemic

Example:
"The world is not safe."

Now let's add the four-dimensional aspects of your brain's map. What were some of the takeaways from these experiences? Draw little thought bubbles coming out of your timeline on the beliefs that were created at that time. What beliefs were planted in the garden of your mind by these events? Did stress in your childhood home lead you to believe, "I'm not worth anyone's time," or "I'll never amount to anything," or "My body is horrible and never does anything for me," or "It's my body's fault for this abuse," or "Something's wrong with me." I could go on and on with examples.

Take a moment now to think about what the take-aways were for you. These takeaways are what you will want to focus on when practicing some of the techniques in this book in an effort to neutralize their charge and create the opportunity to update your brain's software.

Another exercise, for the visual learners out there, is to create a word cloud or a collage of images that represent the "shadow side" or negative takeaways from your past. Next, create a word cloud or a collage of images that represent the "light side" or positive takeaways and moments from your past. Have this ready before the next step. Finally, complete the brainspotting exercise on the next page, starting with the collage of what you want to release and let go of, and at the end, replace it with the collage of what you want to invite into your experience.

THE GARDEN OF YOUR MIND

Growing up, you were a victim of the world around you that was planting seeds in the garden of your mind. As you grow, it becomes your responsibility to weed and rid yourself of the plants (beliefs, ideas, thoughts) that no longer serve your highest good. While creating your brain map's timeline, it can be helpful to listen to bilateral stimulation music in an effort to begin the process of neutralizing, processing, and healing the events that stand out to you.

🌲 EXERCISE: BRAINSPOTTING

🌲 One way that you can neutralize the beliefs, emotional reactions, and intrusive images of your brain map's timeline is through an exercise called Brainspotting. Remember, your brain can be responding to a lot of things all at once because of how brain mapping works. The more negative experiences you neutralize, the less your brain will react to them with current events. Whenever you're watching the news or feeling inundated with any type of intrusive image that is upregulating your nervous system, you can practice this exercise. For now, look at your timeline and choose an event you feel ready to neutralize.

- Choose which memory or series of memories you want to neutralize. Choose something that is below the intensity level of a 6 on a 0 to 10 scale. (If anything is above an intensity of a 6, please only practice this exercise in the company of a trained professional.)
- You can choose one specific image or create a collage of images that go with the same event.
- Hold your hands in front of you and imagine that you are holding the image that you want to neutralize.
- It's often easier to do this with your eyes closed, so you may want to listen to the MP3 and allow me to guide you. 🌲
- Imagine you can see a switch that takes the

image from color to black and white. Switch it to black and white.

- Imagine that you can find a focus dial and turn the dial to make the image(s) blurry.
- Check-in confirmation: You're holding the images in front of you like in a frame, you've changed them to black and white, and you've made them blurry.
- Find the mute button and imagine pressing the mute button so there's no sound.
- Now you're going to move it around your visual field. Don't move your head. Only move your eyes.
- Imagine moving the image(s) into the upper left quadrant.
  - Move it to the upper right.
  - Move it to the lower left.
  - Move it to the lower right.
  - Move it all the way to the left.
  - Move it all the way to the right.
- Check-in confirmation: The image(s) is still black and white, blurry, and muted.
- Shrink the image by 50 percent, so it's half the size that it was originally.
  - Move it to the upper left.
  - Move it to the upper right.
  - Move it to the lower left.
  - Move it to the lower right.
  - Move it all the way to the left.
  - Move all the way to the right.

- ◦ Shrink it again by 50 percent, so it's a quarter of the size it was originally.
- ◦ Move it back and forth a few more times all the way to the left, all the way to the right.
- Now put the frame all the way down at the bottom of your visual field, on the ground so you're looking down on it.
- Imagine that it's on a conveyor belt, and it's moving farther and farther and farther away from you until it's just a speck.
- Now imagine erasing the speck.
- Now bring up an image of someone who's easy to feel love for and one who helps you feel safe and secure.
- Turn that image into color, into focus, and if you want to turn the volume on you may do so, noticing the sounds that help you feel safe and secure.
- Tap on the side of the eye and imagine clicking save. Good.
- Take a deep breath in and open your eyes as you enjoy a nice long exhalation.

How do you feel?

The Brainspotting Exercise, similar to Eye Movement Desensitization and Reprocessing (EMDR), puts the brain on manual mode and guides the brain to neutralize it. I really love this exercise. I find it very effective in removing the charge that some memories can have.

Fear, trauma, and associated conditioning change your perception of who you are and what you're capable of. You want to help your brain return to the truth of who you are.

> **"Truth is what you are. It is your essential nature and being, it is the pure self, the limitless one, the ultimate reality. It is awareness itself. But you have become unaware of the magnificence of your true nature on account of your upbringing, conditioning, and education, which paint a very different picture of who you are— and all of which you believe."**
> **—Mooji**

What I love about this quote is it really helps us identify that you can shift perspective away from what have you been conditioned to believe, how you become conditioned to move or respond or understand depending on your cultural upbringing, your education and knowledge of the body—everything.

Many of us have been taught to push through the pain, play through the pain, have sex through the pain, work through the pain, right? "No pain, no gain" was a common phrase I heard growing up. **When you start to shift your perspective and change the picture of how you see yourself and how you see what's possible, you turn off the faucet of fear.**

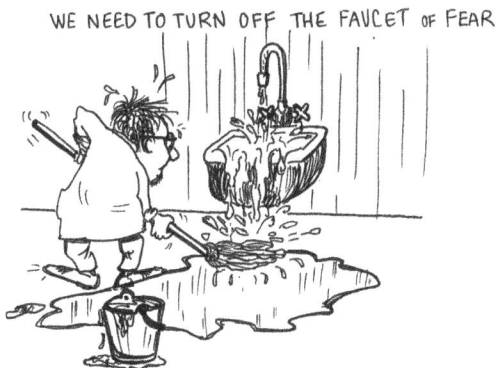

WE NEED TO TURN OFF THE FAUCET OF FEAR

I love this illustration because it clearly demonstrates how many people in chronic pain feel when they're trying to heal with so many different interventions. No matter how much you try to take care of yourself or do what's best, it can feel like it just keeps coming. Do you ever feel that way? When looking at the nervous system and the vagus nerve, you have to think about why the body has a hard time catching up or responding to your interventions. If you don't turn off the faucet of fear, your body doesn't have time to heal itself as fast and as efficiently as it can. If the faucet of fear keeps turning on, you're going to be mopping constantly, and you will start to believe you *won't* get ahead of it. When you're looking at turning off the faucet of fear, you're looking at healing and retraining the vagus nerve.

The Vagus Nerve and the Gut-Brain Connection

The vagus nerve runs separate from the spinal cord (a useful evolutionary development that allows the main organs to continue working even when there is a spinal cord injury), and it roots itself in the pelvic floor muscles—the muscles of the pelvic bowl that hold all of the pelvic organs, such as the bowel, bladder, and reproductive organs. When we're in fight-or-flight mode, the pelvic floor muscles engage, and the entire autonomic nervous system (ANS) goes with it.

As you can see, the lungs are the only part of the ANS that you can gain conscious control over. Everything else you can't consciously control. You can't control your metabolism, your endocrine system, your pupil dilation, your sweat glands, your digestion, or your blood pressure. You *can* control your breath. Therefore, as you calm your breath, you guide your entire ANS into the calm, parasympathetic state. If your ANS is upregulated, it changes the function of your GI system, and vice versa. If you eat something that inflames and agitates your gut, this, in turn, can inflame and agitate your ANS and brain.

Your GI system is your second brain—literally. They are both formed from the same embryonic tissue! You have to calm your gut in order to heal your brain, and you have to heal your brain in order to help heal your gut. It is all connected!

Cytokines, neurotransmitters, and bacterial metabolites can travel to the brain from the gut through blood circulation, thus impacting cognitive function. This is why gut inflammation can, via cytokines, travel to the brain, impacting brain inflammation. The gut can also influence the brain via sympathetic activity communicated by the vagus nerve. Therefore, gut health and ANS health are both vitally important for brain health and optimal ANS functioning.

Gut health is influenced by a myriad of factors. Two strong influences that I focus on in this book are nutrition and emotional health. Food is medicine, and food is poison. Healthy eating and following an anti-inflammatory diet is key to giving your gut a jumpstart at healing. The major inflammatory foods include gluten, dairy, sugar, alcohol, soy, corn, preservatives, and processed food. Once the gut is healed, most people can return to eating these foods *in moderation*. Some will need to remain gluten- and dairy-free for the majority of the time.

Did you know that the gut can create an entirely new lining in only 21 days? How amazing is that?!

Here are some supplements that can improve gut health. I recommend Health Concerns and Pure Encapsulations brands.

- **L-glutamine:** This speeds up cellular regeneration within the lining of the intestinal walls.

- **EnteroMend®:** A digestive enzyme that decreases the inflammatory response to foods.

- **Magnesium oxide:** 250 to 500 milligrams improves GI mobility and serves as a neuromuscular relaxant, which is also helpful for the pelvic floor muscles and nerves.

Due to food having a strong emotional component, it's important to prepare yourself for these changes and allow yourself to take these changes at your own pace. Try not to think of it as an "elimination" diet, because this can be perceived by the brain as "restriction," which creates its own inner panic for many people.

Something that helped me when battling Lyme disease was when my acupuncturist said, "Lyme feeds off of gluten and sugar and dairy. If you want to kill the Lyme, starve it. Don't feed it!" That gave me something to think about on the days when it was really hard to not eat those reliable, emotional coping mechanism foods!

Get creative about how you want to support your emotional health when making decisions to change your diet to support your gut health. Because the vagus nerve connects the gut-brain axis, you want to calm the ANS as often as possible. Remember the pyramid process (see page 23) and utilize bilateral stimulation, breath work, and mindfulness-based stress-reduction techniques.

EXERCISE: MINDFUL JOURNALING

I'm going to guide you through a mindful journaling exercise, which utilizes bilateral stimulation in a unique way. The description is below, or you can listen to a recording. 🌳

In your notebook, write the numbers 1 through 20 down the side of a sheet of paper. On the odd numbers, you're going to notice your thoughts and label them in one or a few words. Imagine you could put all of the thoughts into a file folder. what would you label the folder? That's what you're writing down. Short and sweet is the goal. Sometimes it takes me to number 40 to start feeling relief, but even so, this works every time. The bilateral stimulation comes from utilizing different hemispheres of your brain for each awareness. Your right brain is for your awareness of physical sensations, and your left brain is used for your awareness of your thoughts.* On the even numbers, you're going to notice a physical sensation and write it down. It may look like this:

1. To-do list
2. Tense and painful neck
3. Anxieties
4. Tight chest
5. Chores

---

* Fun footnote: It makes me think of one of my favorite childhood books *I'll Love You Forever* by Robert Munsch when the mother rocks her child "Back and forth, back and forth, back and forth. And sings, "I'll love you forever. I'll like you for always. As long as I'm living, my baby you'll be." That's what you're doing: You're rocking your brain back and forth, soothing it to a peaceful place.

6. Headache
7. Judgments
8. Deeper breath
9. Missing my dogs
10. Tearful
11. Problem-solving schedules
12. Pursed lips
13. Possibilities
14. Smiling
15. Sunny days
16. Relaxed shoulders
17. People I love
18. Deep breath
19. Mindfulness rocks
20. Peaceful

You might feel better already. If so, you can skip the next exercise and come back to it later. Otherwise, let's enjoy some breathwork to deepen the relaxation.

EXERCISE: SLOW BREATHING

With this exercise, you're going to slow down the inhalation and have a long exhalation, and then you're going to slow down the exhalation and have a long inhalation. As with every exercise, note your subjective units of distress (SUDs) level before and after the exercise.

3-Part Inhale

Allow the inhalation to take three parts, breathing into the lower ribs (Step 1), middle ribs (Step 2), and upper ribs (Step 3)

1. Breathe in for 1 count, pause
2. Breathe in for 1 count, pause
3. Breathe in for 1 count, pause
4. Exhale completely
5. Repeat

3-Part Exhale

Allow the exhalation to take three parts

1. Inhale completely
2. Exhale for 1 count, pause
3. Exhale for 1 count, pause
4. Exhale for 1 count, pause
5. Repeat

Lessons from *The Karate Kid*

How can something so simple be dramatically effective? Breathing exercises can feel that way sometimes. Especially when you're in a high level of pain, you might wonder, "How can breathing possibly help me?"

What I love about the old and also the updated version of *The Karate Kid* is how the teacher uses such simple techniques to teach a bigger lesson. In the newer version, when he's training his student, he instructs the kid to practice a really simple exercise of taking off his jacket, hanging his jacket on the pole, taking his jacket and putting it on the floor, picking it up, putting it on, taking it off, again and again and again. In the movie, the kid gets really frustrated and says (I'm paraphrasing), "How am I possibly learning karate doing this?" The teacher responds, "You'll figure it out." It ended up making the kid really strong, strengthening different muscle groups in a creative way. If you haven't seen the movie, I recommend it!

Emotional Freedom Techniques (EFT)

Some of the exercises you'll learn in this book can feel really simple, but they can be dramatically effective. Emotional Freedom Techniques (EFT) is one of those exercises. EFT is a meridian tapping method where you tap (or rub) specific acupressure points on your body. The recent science on EFT demonstrates that it directly stimulates the amygdala to shift out of the fight-or-flight mode and aids in creating more than 72 genetic changes! More than 72 different genes—particularly those related to trauma and fear-based memories—are changing within one hour of tapping. This adds to the body of literature demonstrating that your body will match what you feel and what you say. As you tap on what you feel and what you're thinking, you help your brain process out the old and invite in the new.

Research demonstrates that tapping can eliminate phobias and trauma-related symptoms in as little as 30 minutes without any relapse, even six months later. More than 250 clinical trials have been conducted on the effects of tapping, and it is truly the new "magic wand" in the trauma healing community. Resources on tapping are listed in the back of this book. (See Appendix E.)

I will guide you on how to create your own tapping sequences, which can be most effective. Tons of books and even an app can guide you through the tapping process. **What's most important about tapping is stimulating the points and focusing on your experience.** Tap out what you don't want, then tap in what you do want.

The process for tapping begins with tapping on the side of the hand called the "karate chop point" or rubbing the left side of your chest, called the "sore spot." Then you go through the sequence of points de-

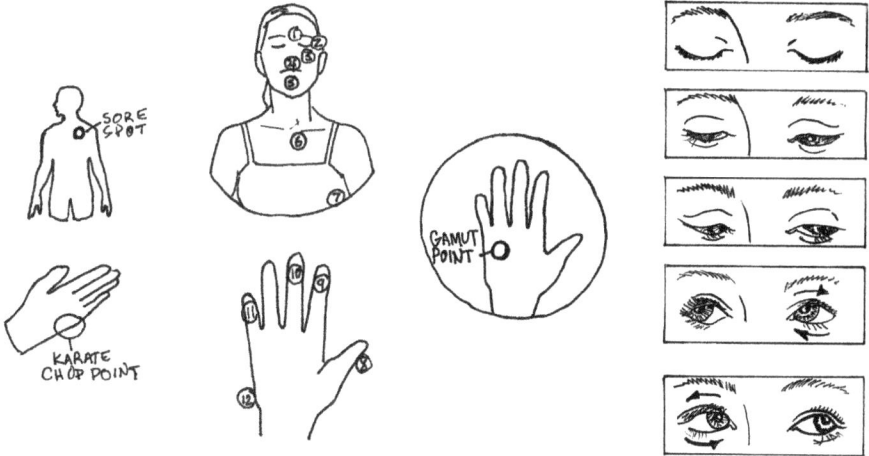

tailed in the image above, including the points on the side of the fingers. Then you'll follow a nine-step process when tapping on the "gamut" point:

1. Close your eyes.
2. Open your eyes.
3. Look left.
4. Look right.
5. Roll your eyes in a circle.
6. Roll your eyes in a circle in the opposite direction.
7. Sing five notes (i.e. the scale or "Twinkle, Twinkle Little Star").
8. Count from one to five.
9. Sing five notes.

Let me talk you through a tapping sequence that's on shifting the perspective of the diagnosis. 🌱 Starting with the side of your hand, think, "What do I believe to be true about my pain and my body because of my diagnosis?" Take a look at the brain map timeline you made earlier and tune into the thoughts and takeaways from your life experience. As you think about your beliefs, perspectives, and fears regarding your pain and associated diagnoses, keep tapping on the side of your hand and say aloud:

- "Even though I have these beliefs about my pain, I deeply and completely love and accept myself."

- "Even though I may not believe that right now, I'm willing to learn how to deeply and completely love and accept myself."
- "Even though I still have these beliefs about my pain and diagnoses, I'm open to a new way of seeing this."

Now, with each new statement, tap on the next tapping point. The order of the points doesn't matter. If a thought comes to mind, feel free to divert away from this script and follow your own train of thought. You might be thinking something along these lines:

- It would take a miracle to heal my pain or change my diagnosis.
- And miracles don't happen for me.
- I don't believe I will be pain free.
- They don't think it's possible for me.
- Even if I get some relief,
- I expect the pain to come back.
- And it always comes back.
- I have this conviction.
- That it's not possible for me to be pain free.
- I would have to make lots of changes in my life,
- And I don't think it would matter.
- I probably wouldn't stick with it anyway.
- Besides, it's not possible to be pain free,
- Why try so hard for something that won't work?
- I want to believe it could be possible,
- Although I'm not there yet.
- I want to believe it's possible.
- But I don't want to be disappointed.
- I don't want to let others down.
- It seems safer to be skeptical.
- I don't want to get my hopes up, again.
- I don't think I could handle the disappointment.
- And the devastation.
- This pain destroys everything in its path.
- It's destroying my ability to believe in healing.
- I don't know what else to do.

- I'm trying this tapping thing,
- Which feels really weird.
- How could this tapping possibly be helpful?
- I'm starting to feel a little calmer, actually.
- Maybe it's doing more than I think.
- Whatever. I'm willing to try anything at this point.
- I sure hope it works.

Great job. Take a moment to read through those statements again. If any of those statements has a charge or intensity higher than a 5 (on a 0 to 10 scale), tap through that sequence again, adding anything else that came up for you during the process.

When your nervous system feels lower than a 5, you're ready to move into the "positive round." Try statements like these:

- What if it was possible to be pain free?
- If I could change this belief,
- How would others react?
- Would they think I made it all up?
- Maybe.
- Maybe not.
- I want to release that, too.
- I want to release caring about what others think.
- It's my body. My life. My experience.
- I want to believe it's possible to heal.
- Maybe it is possible.
- I want to be open to it being possible.
- I choose to allow the possibilities.
- I'm ready to experience new possibilities.
- I'm choosing to accept there could be new possibilities.
- I'm open to new possibilities with this pain.
- I'm ready to let go of my attachment to these diagnoses.
- I don't need them anymore.
- I have a plan now.
- I understand myself more now.
- I'm ready to heal now.

Take a deep breath in through the nose and release through the mouth with a nice, long exhalation.

Great job! That's an example of how you can do tapping around the beliefs that have been created by your life experience. List the beliefs that feel true for you—especially the ones that don't serve your healing journey. Tap on those first and your willingness to shift those. Then tap into the new possibilities, the new beliefs, the new vision.

Tapping literally "taps into" the ANS, calming the vagus nerve, relaxing the entire neuromuscular system. When you tap on both sides of the body, you're also utilizing the bilateral stimulation techniques. Therefore, you're also helping the brain process and neutralize the state-dependent memory and learning that is connected with whatever topic you're focused on.

Something I recommend adding into your tapping sequence is eye movements. When we're in fight-or-flight mode, the brain gets stuck in the right hindbrain, so your eyes will actually stop at the midline when trying to move them. Because the eyes follow the brain and the brain follows the eyes, moving the eyes around helps move the activity in the brain. When you intentionally guide your eyes to go left and right and all around, you manually move the activity around your brain.

Tips for Tapping

Tapping provides support for the brain to process and neutralize the thoughts, beliefs, emotions, sensations, and memories as we acknowledge and feel them. When your brain has this support, it begins to peel off layers, like peeling an onion. This allows you to go deeper and get to the core of the issue.

Once you neutralize the core of the issue, the connected limiting beliefs and uncomfortable emotions and sensations cease. The key is to keep tapping on the issue until it eases into the next layer. You cannot rush this process. Trust the process.

Creating Balance before Tapping

Before tapping, it can help to balance the energy flow in your body along pathways called meridians—similar to having our own fiber optic network.

This exercise also helps balance the activity and circulation in the right and left brain hemispheres. ☥

Do 2 minutes of the Bilateral Crossed-Hands Balanced Breathing Exercise:

1. Seated comfortably, relax and take a deep breath. Place your left foot over your right foot.

2. Breathing in normally, stretch your arms straight out in front of you at shoulder level.

3. Turn your arms, palms facing outward, put your right arm across your left arm, and clasp your hands.

4. Interweave your fingers, closing them with those of your opposite hand, bending your elbows out.

5. Move your folded hands down toward your abdomen, then upward to rest on your chest.

6. Hold this position, relaxing, breathing slowly and steadily.

7. Think the word "balance" and imagine something symbolizing this to you—scales of justice, a carpenter's level, children sitting on a playground teeter-totter—balancing it evenly and perfectly. Focus on how having your perfectly balanced result feels.

Another way to do this is to listen to bilateral stimulation music while tapping.

Calming down the constant checking on your pain's status:

- I'm checking the status again...
- I feel like I need to...
- I feel like I can't stop myself..
- What do I think I'm going to find?
- Will I miss the pain if it's not there?
- Does part of me want it or need it to be there?
- Why do I care so much about if it's there or not?
- Who will I be without the pain?
- If I'm okay with it going away, then I'm okay with not checking on it
- I'm open to not checking the status.
- I know it's healing. I don't want to bother it.
- It feels like watching a water pot boil...the more I watch it the slower it goes...
- So maybe I'll stop watching it...maybe it'll heal faster that way.
- I want my body to heal. I'll let it heal.
- It feels good to let it heal.
- It feels good to let it go.
- I give myself permission to leave it alone for a while.
- I can check on it tomorrow.

SIX MAIN CONCEPTS OF ENERGY PSYCHOLOGY BY MARCUS BARKER, MD

1. The body "remembers" all its experiences in life.

2. A vital energy flows throughout the body. That flow can become blocked, creating a "disruption" and throwing the body/mind out of balance.

3. Accessing and focusing on (but not reliving) an upsetting thought, issue, or event are important to treating the specific problem.

4. Having a troubling thought or problem causes a disruption that blocks the natural flow of energy.

5. This blocked energy can be "reversed" at some point along the meridian. This reversal, which can be corrected, can slow or stop progress.

6. Through a step-by-step procedure involving tapping on acupuncture points, an issue can be resolved or modified.

EXERCISE

Look at the 4-D Wheel you created or your brain map timeline while tapping and see what comes up for you. If you have a therapist who you can do this with, that would be ideal for the more intense memories and beliefs. Having support through the whole process is extremely beneficial. You can also write down your beliefs and record yourself going through the sequence so you can listen to it anytime, anywhere.

"The reason that these same lifestyle changes can prevent and reverse the progression of so many different chronic diseases is that they are the different manifestations of the same underlying biological mechanisms."
—Dean Ornish, MD

The same underlying biological mechanism is the nervous system and the brain. If you can heal the nervous system and the brain, the body will absolutely reverse the majority of chronic diseases and illnesses that you see today. Hundreds of case studies demonstrate that. Dean Ornish, MD, talks about "Lifestyle medicine." The elements of an effective and gratifying lifestyle medicine healing routine include:

- **Deep, restorative sleep:** Sleep is nature's remedy. Nothing else can replace it.
- **Good nutrition:** Organic, low-inflammatory foods, minimal to zero preservatives, minimal to zero processed foods, minimal alcohol and sugar
- **Hydration:** If you're thirsty, you're already a liter behind
- **Regular exercise:** 15 to 20 minutes daily of fast-paced walking decreases chronic pain and inflammation; mindful-based exercise improves brain-derived neurotropic factor (BDNF), which increases neural regeneration and healing.
- **Simple pleasures:** Each and every day, do at least one small, simple, gentle thing that feels good to your body: Watch the sun rise, feel your fingers in the garden, play an instrument, do anything else that brings you joy. Prioritize them in your schedule.
- **Some form of meditation, prayer, or chanting:** Start and end each day with any mindfulness-based stress-reduction exercise. The emotion you fall asleep with is the emotion you will wake up with. Start your day with fresh intentions, and enter your sleep feeling peaceful.
- **Love and compassion:** It's the healing remedy for all living things. Love deeply, completely, and unconditionally. Love is freely given and freely received.

This book will focus on encouraging you to eat well, move more, stress less, and love more! Begin incorporating some of the changes and some of the exercises that you practiced today. Maybe you want to tune into your brain map and tap on your brain map every day during your intentional healing time. Try to increase your healing time by 5 minutes each week until you're up to 20 minutes per day. The more often you calm your nervous system, the easier it will become, and the longer your inner peace will last.

Here are some useful gadgets worth mentioning.

- **Apollo Neuro device:** Utilizes sound frequency to calm the nervous system (discussed more in Chapter 10)

- **Muse device:** Utilizes EEG software to provide neuro-feedback on your brainwaves as you practice various breathing and mindfulness-based meditation exercises. The background music and sounds also change depending on your brainwaves, which engages the reward system in your brain, rewarding you for relaxing and helping the brain click save on this new state of mind.

- **Vibrating massage balls:** I recommend the massage balls by PureRomance.com. Vibration can loosen tight muscles and scar tissue (and bring pleasure!).

- **Mayan abdominal massage:** A gentle approach to increasing circulation and easing pelvic congestion. See the demonstration on my website. 🌲

Chapter 6

The Frequency of Thoughts, Beliefs, and Emotions

Frequency is the hardware of our universe. Frequencies create, destroy, shape, and mold all matter. From the tiny electrons that bounce around our atoms to the large solar flares that can take out satellites, frequencies affect everything and everyone. Therefore, it shouldn't be too difficult to understand that our thoughts, beliefs, and emotions are both created from frequencies and create their own frequencies.

Sometimes we can feel a frequency, such as the sound of the bass in my car when the music is loud. Other times, we depend on our brain and sensory organs to perceive them. Some frequencies can't be perceived with our bodies, so we use scientific instruments to view them or listen to them, such as ultraviolet light, infrared light, or radio waves.

Can you imagine if our senses could perceive all frequencies? Our brains would be overloaded with stimulation, and we wouldn't know what to pay attention to first. I remember a scene in the Superman movie *Man of Steel*, when the young Superman was adjusting to the frequencies of Earth, and his entire system was overwhelmed.

Frequencies surround us and are flowing through us constantly. We must become aware of the frequencies we can gain control over—such as our beliefs and emotions—so we can support and guide our nervous systems to a frequency that feels safe and secure—the optimal frequency for healing.

This chapter is going to explore the effects of our thoughts, beliefs, and emotions on our nervous system and guide you through methods you can utilize to adjust the dial of the frequencies of your mind.

EXERCISE: WIGGLE

Before you read and learn, you want to prepare your body and brain to feel open to receiving, open to learning, open to updating its software. We're going to start with the wiggles! Remember in kindergarten when your teacher would ask the class to wiggle to release some energy before s/he asked you to sit down for learning time? That's what you're going to do now.

- Stand up with your feet hip-distance apart and notice how stiff your body feels. Begin to wiggle.
- Start with your toes and then feet and then fingers. Wiggle and shake them.
- Now wiggle your arms, maybe one at a time or both, whatever you prefer.
- Now wiggle and shake your legs, one a time or both, whatever you prefer.
- Now, allow your legs to relax beneath the knees.
- Allow your arms to relax beneath the elbows.
- Continue with long exhalations.
- Now, release your whole arm from the shoulders down, allowing your arms to hang.
- Do a nice long exhalation.
- Wiggle your legs a little bit more, encouraging your thighs to relax.
- Now allow your legs and arms to fully relax.
- Feel them getting heavier, perhaps you want to sit, recline, or lie down now.
- Allow the support beneath you to do the work.

- Start at the top of your head and invite the muscles around your scalp to release down.
- Allow your hair to hang.
- Allow your brow to soften.
- Soften your eyes and imagine your sinuses opening up.
- Allow your jaw to relax by resting your tongue on the bottom of your mouth.
- Soften your eyes, cheeks, jaw, and tongue, noticing how that softens your throat as you release your jaw.
- Allow your shoulders and arms to hang.
- Allow your legs to be just as they are.
- Now do a long, smooth inhalation through your nose and a long, slow exhalation through your mouth as you say "ahhhh."
- Again, inhale through your nose, and this time exhale with a "hmmmmm" as you hum.
- Allow your body to be just as it is.
- Allow your abdomen and pelvis to be just as they are, not trying to make anything happen because that can be stressful. Simply notice and become the observer of that part of your body.
- If you notice discomfort, find the center of where your discomfort, tension, or pain is right now. Like a slide, imagine that you can send your breath right into the center of it. Just allow it to create a little bit more space. If it's not changing, that's okay. Imagine breathing into the center of it. You're letting your body know that you're here,

you hear it, you feel it, and you're learning how to work with it. You're learning how to respond to it. If your body can have patience with you, you can have patience with your body, knowing that you're healing that relationship between you and your body.

- Great job! Legs are relaxed, feet are relaxed, arms and hands are relaxed. Your scalp and face are relaxed.

- Now, think of someone who's easy to feel love for, and take another breath and allow an extra long exhalation with an "ohhhhhhhhmmmmmm" sound.

- Well done! How do you feel?

As you relax the vagus nerve and you lengthen the exhalation, you also help loosen up your chest simply through the vibration of sound. When you intentionally think of someone who's easy to feel love for, this engages "heart coherence"—an electromagnetic frequency that is emitted from the heart and helps bring your brain into a calmer state of mind. This exercise included energy psychology movements, a body scan, breathwork, and sound healing. Note in your activity log how each of these steps made you feel.

All of this is learning how to tune into your body. You're learning to relax the parts of your body that are ready to relax, and you're holding space for the parts of your body that are maintaining their grip on tension. Allow the tension to be just as it is until you have more time to do some tapping on it or journaling on it. The goal is to calm down the fear response to whatever those sensations are.

---

* As a parent, I recommend the book *Your Child's Self-Esteem* by Dorothy Corkille Briggs.

In your notebook, write this down: **"Everything I'm doing is enough. I am enough."**

A common trauma among all children is learning that they're not enough in some way.* We're going to look at some common phrases that well-intentioned parents, caretakers, teachers, and coaches use. While they are well-intentioned, the child's brain hears it and interprets it very differently. For example, when they hear, "What's the matter with you?" in response to a behavior when they're out of sorts, the child interprets that as "Something is wrong with me. I'm not enough. I'm not doing enough. I'm not making the mark." That belief alone tends to trickle into all areas of life.

If you don't believe that you have the resources or capability to heal, no matter what anyone else says or does, it won't be enough. This is called the "nocebo effect." If you believe something will work, then even a pretend pill will work. It's called the "placebo effect."

Either way, you want to get your head in the game as they say. You need to know and believe on a mental, emotional, physical, and spiritual level that everything you're doing is enough and you are enough. Remember, there is no failure, only feedback.

Thoughts are just thoughts—electrical signals in the brain—until you *believe* them. When you believe your thoughts, it creates an emotional reaction, which engages the autonomic nervous system (ANS). In this chapter, you're going to learn how to challenge your thoughts and look for the evidence of the thought that feels better. The brain always seeks evidence.

Positive thinking in and of itself doesn't work. That's right—I said it. Positive *thinking* tends to create stress if you don't believe it. You can't take this giant leap of faith and say, "Everything is fine" when you're in pain. The body is experiencing the opposite! Sometimes, positive thinking can create high stress in the system because of how invalidating it can feel to your present experience. When you've been in pain for a long time, you can unintentionally get into that place of conviction that it's going to be forever, and usually that's because you're so tired of getting disappointed. If you keep the bar low, you're less likely to get disappointed or feel like you failed or that your body failed you. You can get in your own way if you try to jump to a thought that feels too far away.

Instead, you want to create stepping stones toward the thought of possibility, similar to what you did in the tapping sequence in the last chapter. In that sequence, you talked about being open to new possibilities and challenged some of that conviction that you can get into when it's been so long. Using Socratic logic, you can build a case toward possibility. The stepping stones of Socratic logic may look like this:

- I'm in pain right now.
- I've been in pain before, and it's gone away.
- I've had an injury before, and my body has healed.
- I've healed from cuts and wounds.
- I've healed from colds and viruses.
- Therefore, my body is capable of healing.
- It's probably healing now.
- It feels good to know my body is healing now.

In this chapter, we're looking at tweaking the software of the mind, which we've already started doing when you looked at your brain map and created your timeline. (See Chapter 5.) Take a moment to review your takeaways from your life experiences. If any of them do not serve your highest good (do not feel good and do not bring you closer to healing), those are your red flags in the mind, which increase ANS reactivity.

Over the next few pages, you're going to learn how to recognize the red flags in your mind and how to neutralize them and change them in an effective, sustainable way. The Neuro-Orthopedic Institute (NOI) calls them "dangers in me" or "DIMS." Similarly, NOI labels thoughts and beliefs that create a sense of safety and security "SIMS," which stand for "safety in me." Identifying both DIMs and SIMs are important for healing.

Neuroscience shows that negative stimuli elicit larger responses in the brain than positive ones do, explaining why we tend to dwell more on negative events. We call this "negativity bias," and it holds true even when negative and positive events are of the same magnitude.

In other words, we feel negative events more intensely. So, if you receive one negative comment from your partner and two compliments, you will most likely go to bed thinking about the negative one. Acknowledging your brain's negativity bias is already a great step toward understanding why you dwell on these events, so you can work on how to not do this going forward. Provided that you are not in a direct fight-or-flight state, focusing on the positive can shift your mindset, which will eventually lead to you being less affected by the negative events over time.

Ruminating and dwelling on the negative events will strengthen the neural pathways for negative thinking and worrying. Remember: You have the power to help your brain with tapping, bilateral stimulation, brainspotting, and breathwork. You can also use the power of metaphors and intention, as we use in the 4-D Wheel.

✏️ EXERCISE: JAR OF IDEAS

Write down every negative comment you can remember receiving and place them into a jar labeled "release" or "let go." Then write down every compliment or behavior that helped you feel loved and cared for, and place them into a jar labeled "invite in" or "strengthen." You can do this with all of your thoughts and all of your desires.

This could serve as your mindful journaling for the day! This could provide a source of joyful reminiscing. This could serve as an object to use in ceremony or ritual to burn the pains of the past and decorate the fruitful seeds of tomorrow. You can do whatever you want. It's your job to allow it.

Say this with me now: "I am ready and allowing myself to release what no longer serves my highest good. I am ready and allowing myself to receive all good things coming my way."

EXERCISE: UNINSTALLING DIMS

What are some of the fears or the belief systems that you recognize through doing the brain map exercise that could be playing a role in your pain?

In your notebook, create two columns. Write down your DIMs in one column.

Now, with as many as you can, cross them out and write the new, better-feeling thought in the second column. Even if you don't believe the new script yet, because it needs practice, what does that new narrative look like?

For example, if you write down, "I'm damaged," in the first column, cross that off and replace it with, "I feel out of balance, and I allow my body to return to balance."

Any mental program can be uninstalled, but if you don't intentionally try to install a new one, the old one tends to bounce right back.

Next, use tapping to uninstall the old. Go through your list of DIMs as you tap through the points. Then, once the intensity of the DIMs are lower than a 5, tap through the new script to help install it.

You can help your brain neutralize past traumas and associated thoughts and beliefs. That's what we're going to work on in this chapter. Remember, tapping will change your genetics and can even change the genetic coding from generational trauma. It's really cool, isn't it?

Emotion Follows Thought

When the part of us that worries gets triggered, it's so easy to get sucked into it. In an instant, those worrisome thoughts turn themselves into worrisome feelings. We get caught up in a place where we really don't want to be.

We can spend all our time there if we want, and many people do. They worry about everything, and I think somehow they believe that if they worry enough, it will bring solutions. However, what we really need to do is what is called getting into "receptive mode." Many words have been given to this receptive mode. In some religious and spiritual traditions, such as Christianity, they call it the "still small voice." Others call it being open to an "inner guidance system," "inspiration," or a "wise part of myself." Some call it a "spirit guide" or a "guardian angel."

No matter what you call it, the narrative you hear when you're in "receptive mode" only has good things to say and helps you feel supported. This inner voice is always there, but you can't hear it when fear is guiding you into worrisome thoughts. When you step into receptive mode, you realize those worrisome thoughts aren't true. They are not a reflection of reality. Perhaps they were true in the past, but they are not true today. You can choose to think about something else. You might say, "Well, what else can I think of? It's all that's there."

When you feel stuck, metaphors can help because they get us out of the analytical mind and offer a door into the subconscious mind. 🌳 What is a metaphor you can think of that represents your worrisome thoughts? If you could transform that object into something that represents being in tune with that "still small voice" of intuition—the voice of receptive mode—what would that new object be?

Allow Your Cork to Float

My mentor, Charlie Curtis*, uses the metaphor of a cork floating. He says, "You can take a cork and go down to the bottom of the stream and hold on to the cork for dear life. It's way under water. You can be bound and determined to stay underwater forever. Yet, sooner or later, you're going to forget, and the cork is going to float to the surface. Even if only for a second, you're going to have a moment or period of time during which life is okay again."

When do you forget to worry? Charlie also taught me, "Healing is the process of forgetting to remember that something is wrong."

No matter what's going on, you can catch yourself in the act of limiting yourself (worrisome thoughts and limiting beliefs) and allow your cork to float. If you have 10 things and 9 of them cause you to worry, but 1 of them makes you feel good, focus on the 1 that feels good. If you focus on the 1 that makes you feel good, it will cause those 9 other corks to float, and you'll be free.

If and when this feels difficult to do, return to the tapping exercise and bilateral stimulation to calm the ANS, which will make it easier for your brain to redirect itself to the floating cork.

The Importance of Hobbies

Hobbies are activities that make you feel good—no matter how crappy your day was. You can create origami, a painting, jewelry, or a garden. You can write short stories, construct LEGO, or play an instrument. Do whatever it is that you enjoy. Everybody has something they could put their time into that can make them feel better.

If you've never allowed yourself to start a hobby, now is the time to explore and discover what feels good for you.

---

* If you have the opportunity, one session with Charlie Curtis can change your life. He can be reached at charlieach@yahoo.com. He provides world-class professional training in Mindfulness-Based Cognitive Therapy, Neuro-Linguistic Programming, Hypnotherapy, and Metaphysical Healing.

One of my favorite things that I learned with my roommates in college was to create art by melting crayons. We would sit around the hookah listening to music for hours and create art that we hung all over the walls of our bedrooms. We even got to the point where every square inch of the wall was covered in paper plates covered in melted crayon. Can you imagine that? You don't have to! Here is an example of melted crayon art. 😊

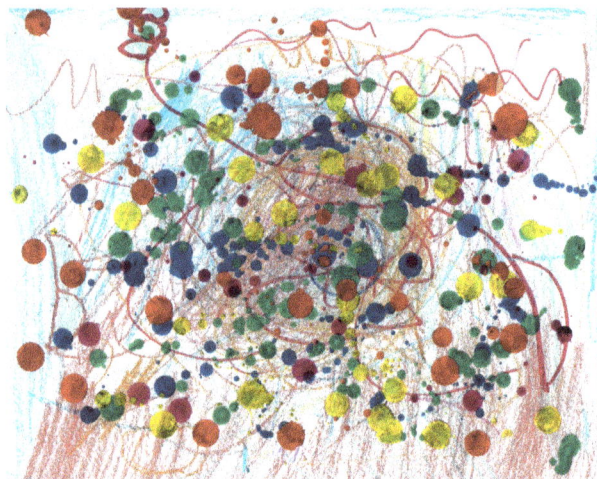

The mind will always amplify what you put into it. If you practice the worrisome thoughts, you're going to amplify the problem. That's going to lead nowhere. If you take the thing that floats your cork and float on that, you're going to feel good and you're going to amplify and strengthen those neural nets.

So what does this mean? All you have to do is focus on things that feel good, and life will get better. **Focus on what feels good. Don't just think about good things. You must *feel* the good things for healing to occur.**

Charlie would say, "You don't have to solve the problems because the problems aren't real." When I was in a lot of pain after my brain surgery, I responded with, "What?! Are you kidding me?! I can't hold my head on my shoulders, and you're telling me my problems aren't real?!" It would make me so mad sometimes. I would feel invalidated—even offended. Of course, that was me in the fight-or-flight mode trance. Charlie wasn't invalidating my current experience. He was invalidating the *meaning and conclusions* the experience was causing me to focus upon.

When you're in a lot of pain, the thoughts and beliefs seem real. They seem real when you're surrounded by conditions. They *seem* real, but they are not a true perception of reality. When you get into that true perception of reality, even just for a second, it will align you into a peaceful place. Even if just for a small period of time, allowing the cork to float will give you the relief that you need to keep going. Therefore, **look for the things that are going to make you feel free**. Things that make you feel free will elevate your consciousness, and they will uplift you. With practice, you'll begin to perceive life from a brand-new perspective. From this new elevation, everything will be okay. Circumstances may be the same for a while because the body—just like a plant—takes time to heal. Either way, your current perception can shift into a better-feeling place. This state is called "solution consciousness."

Allowing Solution Consciousness

When you allow solutions to come into your mind, you now have solutions instead of problems. When you're in solution consciousness, you'll find that all along you were just caught in a narrow band of brainwaves called beta waves. (Think "beta the bully.") Thoughts created by beta waves take advantage of us by pretending they are the only things that exist. For example, when your to-do list is in charge, it tells you, "You have to do these things! It's an emergency! You don't have time for self-care! Self-care is selfish! You don't have time to take care of your physical body. You don't have time to relax. You just have to worry, worry, worry, and work, work, work."

Fight-or-flight mode devotes its entire existence to making sure that you do not take care of yourself. It is fear's mission in life. This mode is problem consciousness. When you're in this mode, you believe you have no other possibility other than to feel stressed. It's exhausting to fight this bully all day long!

I don't want you to fight it. I want you to show it the door and allow it to leave the sacred space of your mind just as easily as it came in. Return to solution consciousness.

When you find something that makes your cork float, all of a sudden you'll be in a different place. There is an abundance of ideas, inspiration, beauty, magic, and wonder in this world. Open yourself up to noticing it. Allow yourself to take that 180-degree turn. Get into the zone of playfulness, creativity, and possibility. When you escape the state that has been keeping you hostage—the state of fear—you'll find yourself having fun.

This is all about getting your cork to float. I love that metaphor. I think it's very accurate. Even just a moment of allowing your cork to float will give you an awareness and perspective shift that you can return to at any time. Some folks I work with will say, "Yeah, but I only felt better for five minutes, and then it was gone. Therefore, nothing works for me." Once again, fear is taking them down the rabbit hole of hopelessness.

EXERCISE: RELAX AND ENJOY THE UNFOLDING

On my website, check out the video "Relax and Enjoy the Unfolding." Try this: Imagine using your arms and hands to hold a bag of corks under water. Feel the tension rising in your muscles. Notice if you're clenching your jaw, if your tongue is pushing against the top of your mouth, or if your brow is furrowed. Notice what it's like to work so hard to keep that bag of corks under the water. Pause.

Now, let it go. Notice your shoulders dropping, your muscles releasing, your mouth opening slightly to let a deeper breath in, and your tongue dropping to the bottom of your mouth. Sigh. Doesn't that feel better?

With all the exercises you've learned so far, which ones help your cork to float? Here's a review of what we've practiced so far:

- Tapping
- Bilateral stimulation music
- Mindful journaling
- Humming and breathwork
- Walking the 4-D Wheel
- Jars of intention

On my busy weeks, I tap and journal throughout my day for two to five minutes at a time. In between activities or clients, I write down whatever the noise in my head is talking about and take three breaths with long exhalations. I use bullet points and summary statements, just like the Mindful Journaling exercise teaches us to do. When I do that, I stay in a good place all day long. I keep reminding myself that life is good. When I write down the chaos and fears, they are not in my head anymore, and I'm back to a place where life feels good again.

Remember: You don't have to do it all at once. You're on a journey. You're on a continuum. If you just spend time every day in that place feeling relaxed, you become open to noticing more and more of those good-feeling observations. Perhaps it's watching birds float on the rising heat waves, squirrels chase each other around the yard, or children smiling as they explore their environment. **No matter what you do, get busy creating the life you want by thinking of your dreams coming true.**

EXERCISE

Identify the one thing that makes you feel good. On my website, listen to the MP3 "Dwell on whatever pleases you."

Grab the Wheel and Steer

Do you want to speed up your return to homeostasis? Then you need to grab the wheel and steer. You wouldn't call a restaurant to order take-out, mumble "food," and expect them to know exactly what you want and where to deliver it. You would call and tell them exactly what you wanted, how you wanted it, and where to deliver it.

Do you think it reasonable to suppose that this life could respond to your thoughts, mental images, emotions, and interactions? Do you think it reasonable to suppose that if you have absolute faith and conviction that something is the truth then you will be certain to experience the results of your desire?

These questions are explored in the study of the "placebo" and "nocebo" effects. It feels good to imagine the power of visualizing and imagining. Sports psychologists, coaches, neuroscientists, and anyone who self-identifies as being successful highlight the importance of not just thinking, but *feeling* the life that you want. If it's true, then grab the wheel and steer.

"The body is its own healer."
—Hippocrates, the Father of Medicine

The following exercises are additional techniques you can utilize to relax and refocus your mind to dwell on whatever pleases you.

◼️▶ EXERCISE: CORE TELECLEARING PROCESS*

Say these statements to yourself or out loud:

1. There is a part of my being that already knows
    (i.e., how to be calm, focused, and ready to learn).

---

* Adapted from the "Ask and Receive" process created by Sandi Radomski, Tom Altaffer, and Pam Altaffer, LCSW, 24th International Energy Psychology Conference.

2. That part of my being is willing to inform the rest of me now.

3. It is doing so now with grace and ease.

4. My mind, body, and spirit are receiving this information.

5. Information transfer is now complete.

How to Have a Stress-Free Day

Here a "stress-free" day is not defined as a day without stress, but a day where you do not allow stress to dominate and control you.

1. Start the day with a few minutes in the morning for a stress-relief technique, such as Mindful Journaling. (See next page.)

2. Anytime you feel stressed, do something immediately to relieve that stress. If you're on the job and can't take a break immediately, you can at least pay attention to your breathing, and even if you don't have three minutes for a three-minute breathing space, whatever momentary time you can get to do nothing, watch your breathing, or simply step back from your life experience and go meta. It will give you some relief. If you have the time and the privacy to do so, steps 1 and 2 work really well. Even if you only have time for steps 1 through 5, it will bring down your stress through catharsis, often remarkably.

3. At lunch or break time, do something on your list of stress-relievers to bring down your stress level. Mindful Eating, Mindful Journaling, and Emotional Freedom Techniques (EFT) are great options for restoring calm and also for putting you back in touch with your goals and dreams.

4. At the end of the day, when you get a chance, do at least a few minutes of some form of mindfulness-based meditation to calm and relax yourself in preparation for the evening.

Another way of understanding the above is that if anytime you feel stress, you do something to relieve that stress, ASAP, your life will improve greatly, and you will experience life as overall peaceful and joyful, not stressful. Mindfulness research bears this out. Mindful Journaling (ideally with bilateral stimulation music) practiced several times a day can accomplish this remarkably easily. Can you imagine what it would be like to experience that?

✏️▶ EXERCISE: MINDFUL JOURNALING

Here's another example of this exercise, which clears the noise out of your head and gets you off to a stress-free start to your day. List the numbers 1 through 20 on a piece of paper. On the odd numbers, write the label of your thoughts or an abbreviated version of your thoughts, i.e., if you are thinking about everything on your to-do list, you're going to write "to-do list." If you're thinking about everything that makes you scared, you'll write "anxieties and fears." On the even numbers, write down the physical sensation you become aware of.

Example:

1. To-do list
2. Tension in the neck, feeling wired
3. So much to do
4. Tension, slight headache
5. Things I should have done already
6. Eyes feel dense and heavy
7. I'm hungry—snack options

---

* Adapted from *Unlearn Your Pain: A 28-Day Process to Reprogram Your Brain* by Howard Schubiner, MD

8. Tension in the stomach
9. Where food comes from
10. Furrowed brow
11. I take life too seriously sometimes
12. Relaxing shoulders
13. Everything gets done in time
14. Stretching the neck, and eyes relax
15. I love puppies
16. Smiling
17. I love nature
18. Deep breath
19. All is well
20. Headache eased. I want to take a nap.

*Free-Writing in Web Form** 🌳

Clustering, or "webbing" is an effective way to brainstorm your way to self-discovery. Clustering allows you to access ideas quickly, using the circling of your ideas on paper to help you more easily go between the right and left hemispheres of your brain, an ability that's key to solving problems.

- On a separate piece of paper, list your current and past stressors.
- Choose one topic/issue from your list of stressors to work on. Write it in the center of a circle. This is the nucleus, or starting point, of your web.
- Set a timer for five minutes.
- Begin to "free associate" on the topic/issue. Open your mind and write whatever thought occurs to you. Write it down in a one- to four-word phrase, then circle what you've written and connect it by a line to the nucleus.
- Now you have two possibilities to prompt your thinking: what you wrote in your nucleus and what you just wrote in the satellite circle and connected to it. Now write down a word or phrase that

represents your next immediate idea/thought, circle it, and connect it to the circle that prompted it.

- Continue this process until the timer signals your five minutes is up. You will end up with a cluster of ideas and thoughts, which may look like a web filling the page.

Guidelines:

1. Keep your hand moving. Write faster than you would normally write in a reflective mood; attempt to dictate your thoughts as they stream across the radar screen of your mind.
2. Don't cross out anything, even if you didn't mean to write what you did.
3. Don't worry about spelling, punctuation, or grammar.
4. Write whatever comes into your mind or comes from your hand.
5. Allow any thoughts and any feelings to be expressed.

On a separate piece of paper: after the web, free-write the feelings that came up during this experience for five minutes. Allow yourself to express any emotions that you might have. Use phrases such as "I feel ___" and "I felt ___."

After five minutes, write three times: "I am relieved to express these feelings."

On a separate piece of paper: After you allow yourself to express your feelings, now process them. Expressing emotions is important, but it is also critical to understand them, gain perspective on them, and begin to move past them. Therefore, in this free-write, make sure to use phrases such as "I see that…," "I realize…," "I hope that…," I need to…," "I want to…," I can…," "I will…," "I understand that…," "I appreciate…," "I wonder if…," "I have learned…," and "I have discovered…"

After five minutes, write three times: "Understanding these issues helps me feel better."

Chapter 7

Heart-Brain Coherence

Electromagnetic waves are emitted from the heart and emitted from the brain. A device called Muse (available on www.choosemuse.com) measures your brainwaves and shows them to you in real time. This provides helpful neurofeedback.

The waves of your brain change depending on your state of mind. If you're in an anxious state, you're in "beta waves." I call it "beta the bully." When you're in beta wave, you're often being a bully to yourself with self-criticism. When you're feeling relaxed, you're close to delta or theta waves.

Your brainwaves affect your heart rate. Changing the brain can help change the heart waves, and changing the heart waves can help change the brainwaves. Some days it's easier to access the mental space; other days it's easier to access the emotional space. In the emotional space, you want to focus on gratitude lists or thinking about someone who's easy to feel love for. Intentionally trying to change your emotional state has a powerful effect on your brain. Its electromagnetic energy can be measured just like I can measure the wattage in a light bulb. Researchers can measure the type of waves that are emitted from the heart and see how that affects the brain.

Try saying these affirmations:

- My body is healing every day.
- My words are law: I feel loved deeply and daily.
- My body is returning to balance more and more every day in every way.
- I feel more whole every day.

- My immune system gets stronger each day.
- I lead with courage in my life.
- I am always aware of the power within me and all around me.
- I believe in myself.

How do you feel when you say these to yourself? Tune into that heart-brain coherence. What does it feel like?

When you can tune into an affirmation or a thought that is believable and accessible, that changes the brainwaves and the heart-brain coherence via the vagus nerve. If you have Muse, notice how your brainwaves change as you read those affirmations.

If you tend to have anxiety, your mental story may sound like this: "Is it working? Am I doing it right?" Your brainwaves are probably in beta mode. If that's happening for you now, start paying attention to your breath. Notice your heartbeat beginning to calm down. Your brainwaves are following your heart's rhythm. Keep breathing slowly with long exhalations. After a few minutes, you may notice yourself dipping into delta or theta.

What I also love about the app that comes with the Muse device is that the background noise changes as your brainwaves calm down. As your nervous system is calming down, and as you're getting into a more parasympathetic or relaxed state of being, the background noise changes from a loud thunderstorm to a sprinkling of rain, and then the birds come out! Of course, they couldn't create an app without a point system, so yes, you get points for every bird. Then your brain wants to hear those birds and get those points—your brain *wants to relax.* Therefore, Muse can successfully create a reward loop in your brain.

There's also a biofeedback device that the HeartMath® Institute offers (https://www.heartmath.org). The HeartMath® Institute has looked at the electromagnetic energy that is emitted from the heart depending on what the emotion is. What's fascinating is that the research is finding this is true across animal species that also feel emotion, including primates. Whatever emotion that you're in, this is the frequency that's being emitted from your heart, which is going to affect your brainwaves.

Heart Rhythms

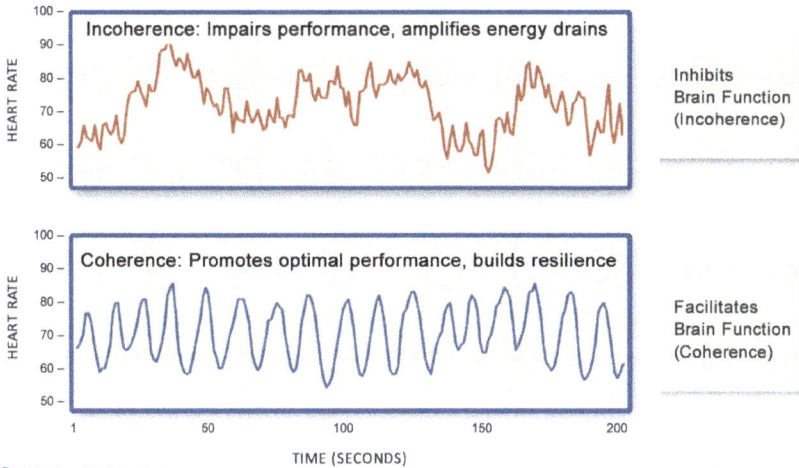

Incoherence: Impairs performance, amplifies energy drains

Inhibits
Brain Function
(Incoherence)

Coherence: Promotes optimal performance, builds resilience

Facilitates
Brain Function
(Coherence)

TIME (SECONDS)

©1997 HeartMath Institute

heartmath.org

*

EXERCISE: STEP INTO THE 4-D WHEEL

There are four different access points to shift the ANS: the mental, physical, emotional, and spiritual quadrants. As you walk around the 4-D Wheel, ask yourself, "Is it easier for me to change my mind? Is it easier for me to change my body posture and breathwork? Does it feel easier for me to access an emotion and shift my emotion? Does it feel easier to access my relationships, such as calling a best friend or connecting with someone who helps me feel loved, nurtured, and cared for?"

Whatever quadrant feels easiest for you, particularly when you're in pain, follow that.**

* Image courtesy of HeartMath® Institute—www.heartmath.org.

** See Appendix C for a list of activities into quadrants.

It's really hard to change your mind when you're in pain, so starting in a different quadrant might be easier for you. Either way, emotions have a frequency that changes your brainwaves and ANS. Emotions have the power to change respiration, heart rate variability, and blood pressure, all of which are really important.

For example, when you're experiencing muscle spasms, you're in the non-coherent state. You tend to be agitated, in a place of frustration, pain, or stress. Maybe you're stressed at work or you're annoyed with your partner. Something like that is going to have the reaction of the pelvic floor tightening, the nerves firing, and the brain having a louder reaction to any of that incoming stimuli. As you shift into a coherent state, as you shift into a state of gratitude or love, or you know an emotion that feels better, all of that comes into play. You calm your mind, you calm your brainwaves, and you literally calm all these different parts of your autonomic nervous system.

The HeartMath Institute's biofeedback device can help, if you want to do it that way. What's really cool is that a lot of different neuro gadgets out there right now can give you feedback to really show you that what you're doing is working, particularly in the beginning stages, when there can be a lot of nervousness and fear of it not working.

Emotion Changes Our Molecules

Here are a few fun photos to bring home the point of how frequency changes molecules, and changes physical things. Many books look at how emotion and the power of words, particularly if we're feeling what those words mean, change molecules.

The Hidden Messages in Water by Masaru Emoto specifically looked at the effect of emotion on water molecules. Keep in mind, inside every living cell is water. The frequency of emotion stimulates movement and the speed of the water's movement dictates how much ATP, or energy, is released from the cell. Low ATP leads to lazy cellular reproduction; high ATP leads to strong cellular production. Lazy reproduction causes us to feel tired and fatigued. It's also what leads to wrinkles on the skin. Strong cellular production leads to reverse aging effects, healing, and increased vitality. We'll look at this again in Chapter 12.

Think about how you talk to your body, how you talk to yourself, and notice how you *feel* when you do. What does your intuition suggest when it comes to how to talk to your body? Would you want shriveled molecules or symmetrical molecules?

To help you remember the answer, think about snowflakes. You want snowflakes in your body. If you want your body to heal as quickly as possible, you have to think about the words and emotions you express toward your body. If you feel like you can't shift that just by thinking differently and rewriting the internal narrative (though this is a great start), then you want to practice tapping or the brainspotting to help get the old story loosened up a bit. Set the intention of, "Even though it's hard for me to believe that my body is healing, I'm willing to believe that it's possible." Just reaching for that possibility gets you closer to healing. Maybe you change the narrative to, "I'm willing to think about feeling beautiful," or "I'm willing to think about feeling purposeful. I'm willing to imagine living a life that feels better," etc.

Ultimately, be kind! Notice your internal dialog, take ownership over the daily script you're practicing, and change it accordingly. Stop practicing the script that was taught to you and trained to you if it causes your body to recoil.

Think about the environment you create around you. We're going to return to this in later chapters when I talk about the power of sound and light frequencies on your nervous system. Take a moment to think about the music, the sound, and the emotion that surrounds you. Do you live in a loving, supportive environment or do you feel stressed and on guard? Are there peaceful, nature sounds around you, or loud, abrupt, disturbing sounds? What are the lyrics of the music you tend to listen to? How does the soundtrack of your life make you feel on a regular basis?

You are about 85 to 90 percent water, so you want to think about how you're affecting your cells by the thoughts and beliefs and emotions you're entertaining throughout the day.

EXERCISE

Fill two jars halfway with rice and fill the rest of the jar with water. Close the lids tightly. Place each jar on opposite sides of the house in different rooms. If you live in a studio apartment, place each jar on opposite sides of the space.

For two weeks, say only mean words to one jar, and loving words to the other jar. After two weeks, you'll notice a major difference between the two jars. The jar you were mean toward will be filled with mold and fungus, and it will look gross. The jar you were loving toward will look the same as it did on Day 1. It will shock you!

I teach this exercise to teachers and parents who deny the power of their words. Once you do this exercise, you'll definitely think twice about how you speak to your body—and to your partner, children, friends, coworkers, and everyone else.

Psychoneuroimmunology

A field of science called psychoneuroimmunology is the branch of medicine that studies the link between your thoughts, beliefs, and immune system. Remember: A thought is just a thought until you believe it. When you believe it, there's an emotional response, there's an electromagnetic response to it, and that engages your immune system, nervous system, and muscular system. You know this because if someone says something that's not true, it can be easy to dismiss it. If it doesn't feel true to you, you can roll your eyes and just forget about it. But if someone says something that matches a negative belief that you also feel about yourself, all of a sudden you have that gut reaction because the gut is the second brain. You might feel tense, emotional, or stressed. You can neutralize this with tapping.

Psychoneuroimmunology paints a clear picture of which neural pathways put the cells of the immune system under the influence of your mind. You don't need to know the detailed science of psychoneuroimmunology. You *do* need to know that this is a branch of medicine that's not taught enough in medical school yet. This branch of medicine demonstrates how your thoughts and your belief system change your DNA, your body's reactions, how your body functions, and how your body heals.

One of the biggest books I've ever read on the mind-body connection and psychoneuroimmunology is *The Irreducible Mind* by Edward Kelly, Emily Kelly, Adam Crabtree, Alan Gauld, Michael Grosso, and Bruce Greyson. It's about 600 pages of phenomenal research focused solely on the power of the mind. I love this particular quote: "The fundamental idea is that anything which produces prolonged stress or other strong emotions leads to biochemical changes. That by affecting systems such as the immune and the cardiovascular system can produce disease, and conversely anything that relieves that stress will reverse those effects and restore homeostatic balance and improve health."

So, that's what you're doing as you calm your nervous system. You're boosting your immune system, guiding all systems into balance. You're improving your health.

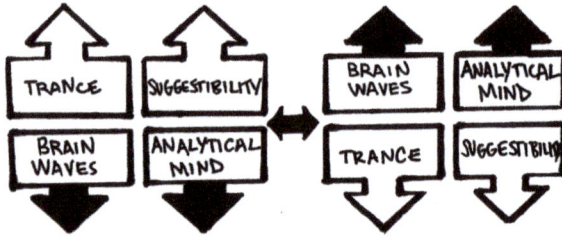

In order for your brain to be open to a new inner narrative, you need to calm the analytical mind. As you can see in the illustration above, when your mind is in a state of hyperarousal, it is not open to suggestion or change. When you're in fight-or-flight mode, nothing is going to change your mind. So that's why you go into tapping, because it calms the system. As you increase the "trance" state, or parasympathetic state of the ANS, you increase suggestibility. In other words, the more you relax, the easier it is to change your inner narrative.

Calming the ANS also brings balance to what the NIH calls the "biofield." The Western world used to think of the chakras* as hocus pocus, but now we're able to measure them and see their effects on the physical body. As we relax and calm the mind, the energy centers in the body align and balance, which also happens when there's heart-brain coherence. This brings homeostasis to all systems in the body. That's when healing happens exponentially faster. So, how do you change your mind?

 EXERCISE

Remember what you wrote in the beginning of this book: "I am capable of learning new skills that benefit my life." Right now, write in your notebook: **"I am capable of and open to changing my mind. Especially if it helps me feel better."** Fast forward to the dream of, "What do I want to think about? What do I want to believe? What do I believe now that I need

---

* Chakras are energy centers in your body. The concept was developed by early Hindus.

to help my brain neutralize through these exercises?" Take a moment to write the answers to these questions.

Next, you're going to create those steppingstones. As you say that statement above to yourself out loud, you're creating a foundation upon which the new narrative can grow. **Make a short list right now of times you changed your mind about something after you gained more information**. This list can include small things or big things. Here are some examples:

- You ordered pasta, and you changed your mind and wanted chicken nuggets.
- You changed songs or radio stations to listen to while driving.
- You switched your undergraduate degree.
- You put back grocery store items.
- You changed plans for dating/changed partners.

By making this list, you're identifying evidence and reminding your brain that you've changed your mind before. If you've changed your mind before, you can change your mind again. As you review the list you made, what motivated you to change your mind? Was it because you thought it would make you feel better? Was it to please someone else? Was it to gain approval? What motivated you? When you think about something that makes you feel better and you do it, the body rewards you by relaxing and being open to joy. Life is more enjoyable when you do what pleases you.

Rethink What You Think You Know

As you think about the process of changing your mind, you're challenging what you think you know. Adam Grant wrote a book called *Think Again* that goes over a lot of really great examples and research on how and why it's important to rethink what we think we know. This is particularly important when you're looking to update your information and change your mental, physical, emotional, and spiritual life experiences. Here are a few important facts that he points out in his book that I want to highlight for you:

- Access to information is increasing at an increasing rate.
- In 2011, you consumed five times as much information per day as you would have a quarter century earlier.
- As of 1950, it took 50 years for knowledge in medicine to double.
- In 1980, medical knowledge was doubling every seven years.
- By 2010, it was doubling in half that time.

The accelerating pace of change means that we need to question our beliefs more readily than ever before. I highlight that because so many times, particularly with chronic pelvic and sexual pain, it's normal to meet multiple doctors who seem to scratch their heads and not really know what's wrong or how to help. That can create a belief of, "If they don't know how to help me, I'm never going to be helped."

Think of someone who died of breast cancer 20 years ago, yet today it can be cured. Western medicine is finally catching up to concepts others have understood for thousands of years, such as chakras, biofields, heart waves, brainwaves, and the power of thought and emotion. EFT has been around for more than 20 years, and just in the past 10 years we've been able to demonstrate *how* it works. Now that we're proving it, we can start increasing access to training and graduate programs.

Why am I pointing this out? **When navigating CPP, it's important to remember that even if you don't have the answer today, you might have the answer tomorrow.** You want to be stubborn about your willingness to keep the door open to possibilities of what can really help heal your system. Think about what you know, what you think you know, things that you know you don't know, and things that you don't know that you don't know.

It can feel scary and overwhelming sometimes to rethink. Rethinking opens the door for grief and regret. If you decide to change your mind about being worthy or being good enough or being smart enough, **you'll probably grieve lost time**. You might say, "Why did I wait until now to change my mind," or "My life could have been so different over the past 30 years had I changed my mind 30 years ago."

Sometimes, even that awareness might hold you back from changing your mind because you can feel afraid of the grief that you might feel if you do change your mind—the grief of lost time and wishing you made these changes sooner. Nevertheless, **you want to be willing to rethink things and challenge what you believe and what you know.** If you listen to that fear response and go back to what's familiar and what's comfortable, you'll only lose more time. What you want to do is help the fear process through the system. Tap on it! This is a great comic that Adam Grant has in his book:

The goal is to always be rethinking and challenging what you think you know. Ask yourself, "What am I really digging my heels in about, and is this making me feel better?" If not, then challenge it.

It's normal to favor *feeling* right over *being* right. Certainly, if you've ever been in a power struggle or relationship dynamic with a parent or a spouse or even a child or a friend, sometimes you can get to that place of knowing that you're wrong, but you unintentionally (and sometimes intentionally) dig your heels in anyway. There's more sustainable empowerment in being willing to rethink things.

Humility, doubt, and curiosity are required to rethink what you think you know. What I love about mindfulness is it introduces you to how to become curious. Mindfulness encourages the curious contemplation of, "What can I become aware of that maybe I wasn't aware of before? What am I feeling? What am I thinking? What are other parts of my body feeling and thinking?"

As you become aware of your beliefs and your thoughts, *insert humility*—a willingness to believe that you could be wrong. Then, begin to doubt your beliefs, and become curious and start to discover the new evidence. All brains are good at finding the evidence for fear. **Stop looking for the evidence that fear tells you is there**! Instead, be curious and discover evidence of the thoughts and beliefs that feel better. You must be proactive about that because your brain will stay in its comfort zone of what it's used to and what it's repeated over several years, let alone several decades. It is going to take intention, curiosity, and discovery to find the evidence of something new.

Metaphors and symbolism can be a powerful way to guide your brain toward change. The 4-D Wheel exercise invites you to identify an object that represents what you want to release and what you want to invite in. I gave you the metaphor of "weeding the garden of your mind." Take a moment to think about the beliefs and thoughts that you wish to release, and that if doing so, would guide your inner narrative to be more kind and loving, and guide your body toward healing faster.

◗▶ EXERCISE: GARDEN OF THE MIND

Write and draw a rendition of a garden metaphor in your notebook. Be sure to draw the pre- and post-healing. For example, maybe you draw a garden filled with weeds and decay, and the post-healing picture is a garden filled with green, vibrant plants, vegetables, and flowers.

Add to the list of DIMs (dangers in me) in your mind that create that fight-or-flight response (and be sure to follow-up as you did earlier with crossing them out and writing the replacement thought in the second column). Identify the DIMs that create a sense of your mind not feeling like a safe place to hang out in. The more you identify them, the more you can clean them out. They usually relate to others' ideas and perceptions of:

- What's right or wrong
- Who you are
- How they want you to be
- Who they want you to become
- What they expect you to achieve
- What they believe you can or cannot accomplish
- What they believe you should or should not do
- What they believe you should know
- What they believe you should think
- Their *responsibility* as a *parent, teacher, friend, mentor*

Other statements that you may hear growing up that get inaccurately or inappropriately translated by your child's brain include:

- Big boys don't cry.
- Be a man, or man up.
- Stop crying, or I'll give you something to cry about.
- It's all your fault.
- Don't be so stupid.
- You don't know what you're talking about.
- Grow up.
- Just wait until your father gets home.
- You never learn.
- Don't be silly.

There are many sayings that you hear growing up that your parents, your teachers, your coaches have passed onto you—and that they, in turn, learned from *their* parents, teachers and coaches. Maybe at the time they were trying to keep you safe; they don't want you to get beat up so that's why they told you not to cry, or maybe they didn't want you to feel weak so they told you to just suck it up. Whatever their intention, it didn't teach you how to tune in and how to deal with insecurities. You learned to stuff it down, and your body is letting you know that you've stuffed a little too much down for too long, and it's time to clean out the house of your mind. The paradox is that the very words that were meant to protect you (hopefully) often have the opposite effect on your way of life.

Return to what you wrote during the exercise above. What you have here is a tapping sequence. You want to tap out the old and tap in the new. There are a lot of different ways that you can work this, but ultimately sometimes just calling it out and throwing the spotlight on it says, "Okay, I'm writing this down to help myself remember that this is *not* what I want to believe because this is not serving me." You might still feel it and, if so, lengthen your exhalation and imagine blowing it away. Calm your nervous system while thinking it, saying it, feeling it, and notice the strength of it fading. As you calm your brainwaves, you're able to reprogram your mind.

> **Worrying is using your imagination to think about what you don't want. Instead, use your imagination to think about what you *do* want.**

As you write down what you do want in the second column, you're intentionally giving yourself permission to imagine a life that could feel better. Ask yourself, "What if I believed this new narrative? What might that be like?" Can you use your imagination, even if you don't believe it yet? Can you still intentionally choose to imagine what it's going to be like when you do? **Imagination is key.** When you're reviewing your DIMs, ask yourself, "Is this supporting me in my goals? Is this an opportunity to grow? Is this enhancing my life?" If the answer is no, then you want to cross it out and choose something else.

Byron Katie, an American author and inspirational speaker on self-healing at www.thework.com, provides an approach to challenging unhelpful beliefs utilizing four questions:

1. Is it true? (Usually if we're in fight-or-flight mode, the ego comes in and says, "Yes, it's true. I know that I'm not good enough, or I know that I'm not that.") Then we move onto the second question.

2. Can I absolutely know that it's true? ("Well, no, I can't be absolutely sure that my body is incapable of healing.")

3. How do I believe, how do I feel when I believe that thought? ("Well, when I believe the thought of I can't heal/my body won't heal from this, I feel pretty crappy.")

4. Who would I be without that thought? (Commonly, this question inspires a deep breath and a sense of, "Oh, I would feel so much freer." In this moment, allow your imagination to go to a place of, "Wow, what would that be like if this program was not running in my mind?"

Embrace that breath of fresh air, that sense of possibility, that sense of, "Wow, I can give myself permission to think about the new narrative." You want to take control. Exercise your right to think for yourself rather than letting your mind control everything that's going on. You want to decide what you want to hear and what sensation you want to focus on. Once you've written down some of your DIMs, you can use your body to shift the feeling. Try the next exercise.

EXERCISE

When thinking of the DIMs, close your body, close your eyes, pull your arms and legs into a ball, and hold—embodying what it feels like when the mind holds on to beliefs that don't feel good—holding on to all of the convictions that pain has convinced you of. Breathe in and hold. As you release your breath, open your body as wide as you can. Open your arms and your chest, lift up your face to the sky and open your eyes. Repeat this alteration—using your body as the metaphor of feeling "closed off" then "open to change."

You're doing a few things here. One, you're moving your body in the way that your mind is acting. When you physically move your body in the way of what you're thinking and what you're wanting, it gets the whole system engaged. "Yes, this is what I want. I want to feel open, I want to feel powerful. I want to feel possible." When your body is closed, you may think, "I don't want to feel like this. This is exhausting. This is where I've been for years." Then you open your body again and say, "Yes, this is what I want to feel." As you close your body and open your body, you're *embodying* what you're saying—helping it become more visible and kinesthetic, which can help it become more obvious as to why you want to change your mind. Remember the tiger story. Imagine him pacing back and forth, back and forth in that cage. Now, imagine feeling that open field. Say to yourself, "I am no longer in this cage. I am no longer trapped in the cage of fear." **As you move your body, you move your mind.**

EXERCISE: TAPPING

Start on the side of your hand, then go through the points with each statement.

- Even though these beliefs may be part of my pain, I'm willing to think about rewriting these thoughts and noticing how that helps ease my pain.
- Even if I believe that I can't change these thoughts or my pain, I'm open to changing my mind about that.
- Even though this feels really hard, I allow myself to do it anyway, because why not.
- This feels really hard.
- These thoughts have been with me my whole life.

- When I look at my DIMs, my brain map feels overwhelming
- It feels like too much.
- How can I possibly rewrite that whole narrative?
- I feel this tension in my body, and maybe it's fear.
- Fear of change, fear of grief.
- Fear of realizing I have more power than I've allowed myself to have in the past.
- I recognize that I'm afraid of change.
- At the same time, I want change.
- I'm realizing the paradox in my mind.
- It feels good to recognize all these different pieces of the puzzle that I can change.
- I don't need to change them all now.
- It doesn't need to take a lifetime to heal them, either.
- I'm willing to take things at my own pace.
- I'm willing to exercise my right to think for myself.
- I'm willing to practice creating my own narrative.
- Even if I can't change the original story.
- I can write a new one.
- At least I have a different channel to tune to.
- It feels good to know I have a new narrative that feels better.
- I'm ready to choose the new narrative.

Keep tapping as you follow the stream of thoughts in your mind and the emotions arising as you read the DIMs and the replacement thoughts.

REBT

Rational Emotive Behavioral Therapy (REBT) offers us another approach that can serve well those who have analytical minds and those of you who like to complete charts and worksheets. I changed the approach slightly, but it looks like this:

A Activating Event	B Belief	C Emotional Consequence	D Dispelling Belief	E Evidence for New Belief
Burning in genitals	It's not going to ever go away.	Fear and anger	My body is capable of healing.	Healed from cuts Healed from wounds Healed from colds Healed from surgery …. Memories of healing … Evidence the physical human body is capable of healing

Column A stands for "activating event." What triggered you? Column B stands for the belief that it triggered. Column C is the emotional consequence. What is the emotion that this belief creates? What is your emotional reaction to that triggering event and belief? Column D stands for dispelling belief, or the new belief. What do you want to believe instead? Column E stands for evidence for the new belief.

Our mind is like Google—it will find answers to anything you ask it, but it doesn't necessary mean it's the correct answer. If we ask the mind, "Why can't my body heal?" we're going to get answers we don't like! Noah St. John wrote a great book called *The Book of Afformations*, in which he discusses the need to *form* the correct questions and statements if we want the mind to help us find the evidence for it. See the example here and take a moment to create your own chart.

✏️▶ EXERCISE: CREATING YOUR SIMS = "SAFETY IN ME"

It feels easier to change your mind when your system is feeling safe. What helps you feel safe? Return to the list you made earlier in your notebook. Sometimes it's images, people, a memory of when you felt safe, an environment. When identifying your SIMs, your goal is to create a place of sanctuary where you can go to help yourself feel safe. Here are some ideas that you can add to your list of SIMs:

- Understanding your pain
- Remembering when your body healed in the past: What did you believe when your body was healing?
- Having a strong support system
- Being aware of scientifically proven paths to recovery
- "There is light at the end of the tunnel."
- Gentle, loving touch
- Cuddling with pets
- "It's a bend in the road, not the end of the road."
- Visiting a happy place

There are many doors to safety. In Appendix C, there is a meditation called "A guided visualization to your perfect place. 🌳 It guides you through a visualization to think about a time when you felt safe and relaxed, and that could be a helpful visualization if you're looking to really work on challenging old thoughts and belief systems, and shift your nervous system. Remember the order: (1) calm your system, (2) reprogram your mind.

The Popular Vote Wins

Neurologically, the more you have a specific thought, the more that neural net gets strengthened. That's why those old thoughts and those old belief systems feel so stubborn—like getting rid of poison ivy! They come up easily and automatically because those are the ones that have been practiced the most, and therefore, they have the most roots. The more you can intentionally redirect the thoughts and practice the new narrative, the more you're strengthening those neural nets, and the easier it's going to be to change the channel. In your mind, the popular vote wins! How are you casting your votes?

The STOP Procedure

The STOP procedure: "S" stands for **stop**, "T" stands for **take a breath**, "O" stands for **observe**, and "P" stands for **proceed**. If you can't find 5 or 10 minutes yet in your life to focus, although you're setting an intention to do that every day, at least take a moment to stop, breathe, notice what you're feeling, notice what you're thinking, notice what's happening in your body, and then proceed with curiosity and interventions.

Ask yourself: "What do I want to do about it? Do I want to change my thought? Do I want to change what my focus is? Do I want to do a stretch or move? What's the intervention that I want to do at this moment? Do I want to do something about it? If so, what do I want to do about it?"

Hopefully, you are starting to feel that you are building up your toolbox of things that you can do, rather than feeling, "Well, I'm aware that there's pain, and I'm aware that I'm thinking about this, and I'm aware that I'm in fight-or-flight mode, but I don't know what to do." I've given you a lot of different ideas and things that you can do right now. You want to insert an intervention and try to change the channel of your mind as much as possible. If you were driving in a car listening to a horrible song, would you keep listening to that song or would you change the station?

The most important diet is the diet of negative thinking and fear-based daydreaming. **The mind is the architect, and the body is the builder.** You're responsible for providing the illustrations of what you want. Chronic pain is a habit within the brain and the nervous system. Both are capable of healing in biology and function within 30 days.

Creating Effective Affirmations

You need to feel it to heal it. Remember the frequency of thought and the frequency of emotion. If you're not feeling it, it's harder for your brain to click save. Tapping can shift the fear. Another key to effectively creating affirmations is to have the language that works for you. You want to create affirmations in a way that feels accessible, that feels believable. Using present, active tense is also key for your subconscious. You don't want affirmations to be in the future tense, such as "I will heal." That accidentally tells your subconscious that it won't happen until sometime in the future. You want your subconscious acting on the positive affirmation *now.* Here are some examples:

- I'm finding balance.
- I'm willing to think about the possibility.
- I'm open to believing my body can heal.
- I'm ready to notice improvement, and improvement is possible for me.
- I am excited to get better.
- I am allowing my body to heal.
- I have all the resources I need.
- I am watching in amazement as my body heals and transforms.

- I am allowing myself to have amnesia for memories that no longer serve my highest good.
- I am feeling supported every step along the way.
- I am allowing my body to find its new equilibrium
- The way to healing is already within me. All I have to do is change the stream of my mental thoughts and imaging. I let my vision be on perfect health and vitality.
- It is normal to be healthy. There is within me an innate principle of harmony. I believe in perfect health, prosperity, peace, and wealth.

These little language tweaks help healing feel possible.

PROGRAM YOURSELF FOR PEACE, HEALTH, AND PLENTY BY CHARLIE CURTIS*

Guide to filling out the form (on page 154) to prepare for the exercise:

1. Identify the issue and your negative thoughts about step 1.

2. Select a goal image (what you want to achieve) and an affirmation (what you would say to yourself if this goal were already true).

3. Select "yes set" images and ideas that feel wonderful when you think about them, are absorbing to think about, the kind of thing that would make a good daydream or reminiscence.

4. Sensory awareness is a simple way to induce meditation that feels wonderful and is very healthful for the body. Write down several sensory memories you can recall, or as an alternative, select several sensory elements from

your present experience that will be pleasant to meditate on.

5. Shift your emotions to a more positive place using the format below.* This only takes a minute, makes you feel much better, and the rest of the exercise becomes much easier.

6. Dwell on your sensory images to relax into a meditative state.

7. Now go through the "yes set" images on the form, and then your goal image and affirmation, and notice how much better you feel.

*Adapted from "Moving Up the Emotional Scale" exercise in *Ask and It Is Given* by Jerry and Esther Hicks, published by Hay House.

Shifting Emotions to a More Positive Place

The following is a list of emotions written in a particular order, from highest to lowest frequency. Start with the lowest emotion that you feel. Create a sentence expressing what you feel with that emotion. Then slowly move up the emotional scale, finding the next emotion you are feeling, and write a sentence. Continue this until you get to the highest frequency emotion of love and gratitude. End with identifying someone or something that you easily feel love and gratitude for.

Love, gratitude, joy, passion, trust, enthusiasm, clarity, freedom, intuitive knowing, empowerment
Happiness, optimism
Hope, contentment
Pessimism, boredom
Frustration, irritation, impatience
Overwhelm, worry, disappointment, doubt
Blame, anger, control, self-righteousness

Hatred, rage, envy, jealousy, obsessiveness
Guilt, insecurity, unworthiness, self-sacrifice, feeling trapped or controlled
Fear, grief, depression, disempowerment, despair

Example of shifting emotions to a more positive place:

- This goal seems impossible. (despair)
- I'm angry about my slow progress. (anger)
- It just seems like it's taking forever. (discouragement)
- It is true: Sometimes it does seem like a possibility. (hopeful)
- I am going to do this. (optimism)
- I am looking forward to this. (positive expectation)
- It's going to be wonderful when I heal. (enthusiasm)
- It feels good to know I'm healing and returning to the life I love. (empowerment)
- I feel grateful for every moment with my son, who I love so deeply. (gratitude and love)

EXAMPLE FORM: Program Yourself for Peace, Health, and Plenty

1. Identify the issue and your negative thought about it:
   Issue: I have had insufferable pelvic/sexual pain.
   Negative thought: I am never going to heal and no one can help me.

2. Select the goal image/affirmations in step 6, the "yes set" images and affirmations in step 5 and sensory experiences in step 4.

3. Shift your emotions to a more positive place using format above.

4. Dwell on sensory images to relax into a meditative state:
   a. I enjoy sitting with my feet in the lake.
   b. I enjoy sleeping and waking up rested and refreshed.
   c. I am listening to the birds while lying in a hammock.

5. Slowly review the "yes set," enjoying the pleasant process:
    d. I had a moment of relief during breath work.
    e. My body has healed from injuries before.
    f. I love being with my best friend.
    g. I enjoyed watching the sunset yesterday.
    h. I really enjoy watching my favorite TV show.
    i. I really enjoy walking in the woods near the creek.
    j. I love listening to the ocean waves.
    k. I love hearing a child giggle.
    l. I enjoy sipping my favorite tea.
    m. I feel joyful when I am playing with my animals.

6. Ponder the goal from this lighter and more positive inner state:
    n. Goal Image: <u>Moving and living the life I love pain-free and feeling strong.</u>
    o. Affirmation: <u>My body is an incredible healing machine, and I allow amazing people to show up to support my progress.</u>

How do you feel now about the goal? "I feel MUCH better. My goal seems possible now. I'm so glad I did this!"

EXERCISE: CREATE A MANTRA ROPE WITH 21 KNOTS*

Find a rope or string to use, like a shoestring. Tie 21 knots in it. Having a physical mantra rope can be very useful to help your brain focus physically and visually. You can feel it, similar to meditation beads. It helps keep you focused on what you're wanting to focus on and what you're wanting to practice in your mind. Why 21 knots? Because 21 seems to be a magic number for the brain and the body. They say it takes 21 days to break a habit and start a new one. It takes

* Adapted from Charlie Curtis (2012) with permission.

21 days for the GI system to have a completely new lining, which is why if you do an elimination diet for three weeks, that's extremely beneficial. It's pretty amazing that your body is able to completely renew itself within three weeks, is it not?! It only takes 21 to 28 days for our brain's hardware to heal. When you are calming the nervous system and practicing these mindfulness exercises, 21 is a magic number. When it comes to mantras and affirmations, saying it 21 times helps the brain click save. Going through 21 knots and stating your affirmation 21 times will only take about 30 to 60 seconds. Something else I love about a mantra rope is that it's a physical reminder to practice mindfulness. It's a physical reminder to tune in and ask, "What am I thinking? How am I feeling right now, and do I want to do something about it?" Having the rope in your purse or on your desk can be a visual and kinesthetic reminder.

The intention of sprinkling these exercises throughout the day is to demonstrate to yourself that it doesn't have to take very long to reroute your nervous system and reroute your brain. Placing the mantra rope on your table can be useful to bring mindfulness and healthy intentions to every meal. An affirmation that I love to have (especially when I'm eating junk food) is, "Everything I put in my body turns to health and happiness."

If words have power, if thoughts have power—which you know that they do because the science demonstrates it—how can you set an intention before you take medication or supplements or eat a meal? What do you want this medication to do? "I allow this medication to help me heal," feels better than, "I hate taking meds, and now this might not work, and I'm in fear because I'm thinking about the side effects." If that's what you're thinking, then you're in fight-or-flight mode, and your food is meeting an anxious stomach. That's going to change how your stomach digests the food and how your system metabolizes the medication.

There are many different moments and opportunities throughout your day to practice mindful moments, positive affirmations, and positive intentions. Even when drinking a glass of water, look at the glass and say a prayer or set an intention, such as, "I allow this water to clear my system of inflammation and toxins." Remember the water molecules and how they change with emotion and words. You want to help your body receive food in the most healthy, vibrant loving way possible.

Whether you make a rope with 21 knots to remind you throughout the day to be present and to be kind and loving and intentional with yourself, or whether you do it every time you have a meal, all of these are opportunities for being intentional and kind to yourself because that's really what mindfulness is all about.

Wellness that is being allowed or the wellness that is being denied is all about the mindset, the mood, the attitude, and the practice thoughts. There is not one exception in any human or beast, because you can patch them up and they will just find another way of reverting back to the natural rhythm of their mind.

Treating the body requires treating the mind.

Deep fears and deep beliefs in your brain and in your subconscious are there, and they will continue to be there until you neutralize them. When the nervous system is upregulated for a prolonged period of time, the body gets sick; it's what happens when the body is out of balance. Next, you'll learn more about one of the most healing exercises in the literature today: mindfulness.

Chapter 8

Mindfulness

"Mindfulness means paying attention in a particular way: on purpose, in the present moment, and nonjudgmentally."
—Jon Kabat-Zinn

Mindfulness Creates Trust

Through mindfulness, you create trust. You create a trust between your mind and body because you're tuning in and you're not dismissing it or ignoring it. You're asking yourself throughout the day, "How can I nurture myself? What is my body needing? If I'm thirsty, am I getting a glass of water? If I'm sitting too long and I need to move my body, do I allow myself to stand up and move around? If I'm reading this book and I need to go to the bathroom, am I pausing and going to the bathroom?" How are you listening? How are you helping your mind change channels to a soundtrack that feels better?

An influential moment in my life was when I met Jane Goodall. Her work and story inspired me to earn my degree in Sociology and Anthropology. She inspired me to be curious, and most importantly, to be patient. Jane Goodall offered chimps not only a deep trust, but also patience and persistence. Jane Goodall did not walk into the forest and the chimps automatically trusted her.

Of course not! The trust took years. Improving the trust within your own mind-body connection does not need to take this long, but it's that same concept of "good things takes time."

If you've spent a lifetime distrusting or not listening to your body, pushing through the stress, pushing through the pain, following that "no pain, no gain" concept, your body doesn't trust your mind, and your mind has stopped trusting your body. The more often you tune in and notice what your body and heart are asking for, the stronger the trust will become. The stronger the trust between you mind and body, the faster your body will respond to your interventions and relax more deeply. Your body says, "Oh, you're listening now, so I don't have to yell in order to get your attention." This is the trust that we're going for between your body and mind.

Default Mode Network: Your Childhood Narrative

When you look at someone's brain under a functional MRI scan who is in fight-or-flight mode, you see a part of the brain lighting up called the "default mode network," which is the medial frontal cortex. This is where the narrative of your childhood lives. All the seeds of beliefs that were planted while you were growing up, particularly before age 11, get activated. Those are the beliefs that tend to spin around, including, "I'm not important enough. I'm not good enough. I'm not lovable. I don't have what it takes." When you hear that narrative start to play, remember that it's only playing because this part of your brain is lighting up and playing the movie soundtrack. You can say to yourself, "Thank you, brain, for trying to keep me safe. I'll take it from here." Then change the soundtrack.

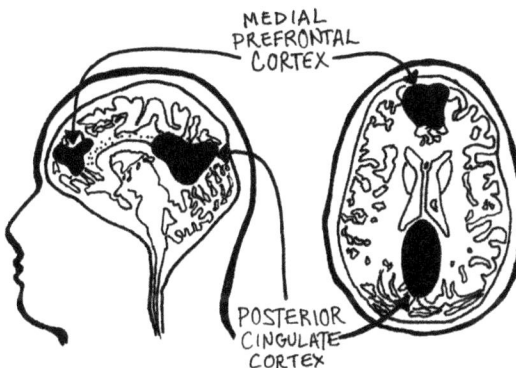

MIDLINE AREAS of the DEFAULT MODE NETWORK
MEDIAL PREFRONTAL CORTEX
POSTERIOR CINGULATE CORTEX

THIS IS WHERE OUR CHILDHOOD NARRATIVE LIVES.

Step Behind the Waterfall of Life

Metaphorically, you can imagine you're standing underneath the waterfall of life. Mindfulness helps you step back, even if you can't change it. Stepping back may not be able to change the waterfall, but you can get relief from stepping behind it. Step one is recognizing when you're standing underneath it. Step two is choosing to step behind it. When you try to step back and it doesn't work, start tapping. The bilateral stimulation of the music by Jeffrey Thompson can help, too. Going on a walk can help. Many different things can help you step behind the waterfall of life. Even if you can't change the narrative today, you can at least recognize that it's playing and choose not to believe it. You might not be able to change the channel, but you don't need to keep watching it. How can you gain a little bit of space from it? You guessed it: mindfulness. The practice of mindfulness is what can help give you the ability to make that space.

Dr. Siegel's Wheel of Awareness

Dr. Daniel Siegel has a phenomenal book called *Aware* in which he detailed his "Four Circles Bright Minds Program" and his recommended "Wheel of Awareness." This is his approach to mindfulness and the research behind the power of mindfulness on physical, mental, emotional, social, and spiritual well-being. He recommends starting with paying attention to the five senses—similar to what I started with in this book, utilizing the 4-D Wheel and the "Quick I Spy" exercise that follows on page 170. With the hardware changes that happen with chronic pain and trauma, tuning into the interconnection or the mental activities or the bodily sensations can be difficult. When you start with the five senses, it brings your attention outside of yourself and into your environment, which helps your nervous system create a sense of safety and security. This is a great foundation to start from.

Then he recommends moving your awareness into bodily sensations. For example, this includes focusing on your breath, practicing progressive muscle relaxation exercises, and tuning into what you're sensing physically.

Then he recommends moving into mental awareness, such as the DIMs you identified earlier. Finally, after you have practiced the above approaches to mindfulness, he recommends practicing the awareness of interconnection. The 4-D Wheel helps with this, as it includes the spiritual quadrant—the quadrant of connection and disconnection.

I agree with Dr. Siegel's approach to mindfulness practice, especially when it comes to navigating pelvic and sexual pain. When you're in a pain flare, go back to the five senses. When you're out of a flare and feeling more calm, that's when some of these other mindfulness practices are going to feel more accessible and effective.

WHEEL of AWARENESS

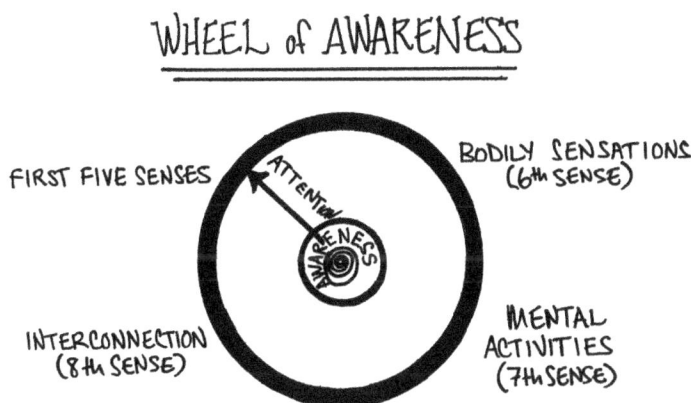

FIRST FIVE SENSES — ATTENTION — AWARENESS — **BODILY SENSATIONS (6th SENSE)** — **INTERCONNECTION (8th SENSE)** — **MENTAL ACTIVITIES (7th SENSE)**

Mindfulness: Compassionate Curiosity

Angus Fletcher is a neuroscientist and a fascinating fellow. I had the pleasure of meeting him at Chautauqua Institution in the summer of 2021 when he did a talk on artificial intelligence. During his lecture, he stated, "Curiosity is the only way to change your mind and open your mind to influence. Otherwise, the brain only collects information that matches what you've already decided. Information delivery does not change minds in and of itself."

Remember back to Adam Grant's research demonstrating the need for humility, doubt, and curiosity in order to discovery new perspectives? Mindfulness invites that opportunity to be curious. Instead of asking, "Body, what is wrong with you?," choose the kind, loving approach: "Hey, body, I can tell you're upset. What can I do for you? What do you need from me?" You want to be curious. When you're curious, you can feel empowered about what can be done to help.

The definition of mindfulness is the ability and the practice of becoming aware in the present moment, the here and now, with a compassionate presence.

> **"We don't see things as they are.**
> **We see things as *we* are."**
> **—Anais Nin, 1961**

You perceive things through the filter of your brain map. Mindfulness helps you become aware of that filter with a compassionate presence. Mindfulness transforms distress into curiosity, even in the face of dissonance, threat, loss, and doubt.

Tara Brach offers us her "RAIN" acronym, which is a mindfulness twist to the STOP protocol. "R" stands for **recognizing** what is happening. "A" stands for **allowing** the experience to be there just as it is. "I" stands for **investigating** with interest and care, becoming passionately curious. "N" represents **nurturing** with self-compassion and non-judgment. Here's an example of what applying the RAIN approach may look like for you:

- I recognize my bladder urgency and pain.
- I allow the experience to be there. (If you remember in previous chapters we talked about the definition of acceptance and how that doesn't mean I'm OK with it being there. I'm not saying that I want it. I'm just recognizing what's happening in this moment and allowing it to be just as it is.)
- Then I investigate it—I become curious about it. "Is it nerve pain? Is it a muscle spasm? Is it gas? Do I need to pee or is it just my muscles spasming? You know what, let me investigate this a little bit more. Where does the pain start? Where does it end? What's happening in the rest of my body?"
- Finally, we get to nurturing it. "What am I going to do about it? If I was going to be loving to myself, what would that look like? If I

was talking to a friend and they were telling me these things, what would I recommend to them? If I was talking to my child, or if my dog was whimpering, how would I respond to them?

- Summary: You're recognizing what's going on. You're allowing the experience to be there. You're investigating it with curiosity, and you're offering a nurturing response. Doing something about it is increasing that trust between your mind and your body.

Take a moment to practice the RAIN protocol now. Then, take three long breaths, focusing on lengthening the exhalation. How was this response different from your common responses to your body's signals?

Active Mindfulness

If you find meditations difficult, you need to start with "active" mindfulness. Active mindfulness requires your attention in the present moment as you actively participate in an activity. Don't worry, you don't need to start skydiving. ☺ As you heal the brain and you practice mindfulness, meditating becomes easier. Here is a list of active mindfulness practices you can explore.

- Breathwork
- Singing
- Progressive muscle relaxation
- Mindful eating
- Playing "I Spy" with all five senses
- Swimming
- Creative arts
- Sensate-focused touch
- Mindful exercise, such as yoga, Qi Gong, and Tai Chi
- Playing an instrument
- Playing Ping-Pong
- Playing "red light-green light" game with children
- Playing "Simon Says"
- Brushing your teeth with your non-dominant hand
- Mindful walking

All of these exercises are really about retraining that part of mind to be in the present moment. A simple definition of mindfulness can be: **Pay attention and be nice.** Set an intention to do just that: Pay attention to yourself and be nice.

Empathy versus Compassion

Tania Singer, a neuroscientist and a social scientist, focuses her research on what's happening in the brain when someone is feeling empathy compared to when someone is practicing compassion. She discovered that **empathy and compassion are two different neural circuits in the brain**. Interestingly, empathy is the same circuitry as pain, while compassion is the same circuitry as pleasure.

Empathy comes naturally to most of us, thanks to our "mirror neurons." Our mirror neurons initiate our brains to light up in the same way and in the same places that someone else's brain is lighting up. It creates a "mirrored" experience. If you are watching someone who is feeling sad, you may notice yourself feeling sad. If you are watching someone who is feeling happy and smiling, you may notice yourself mirroring their smile and feeling happy. The most obvious examples are when you are responding and reacting to TV and movies, and when you're reacting to your best friend venting about work or telling you an exciting story. Empathy is a two-way street—you're literally "in the brain soup" of the story you are listening to.

Meanwhile, compassion is a one-way street. Compassion is sending someone a feeling of loving-kindness and wishing them comfort and peace.

The best way I can think of to describe the difference between these two is through a story. If you see someone drowning and you jump into save them, but you start to struggle and drown with them, that's empathy. You're experiencing what they are experiencing. If you see someone drowning and you throw them life jackets, ropes, and rescue gear, but you choose to stay out of the chaotic waters, that's compassion. When we are in a state of empathy—a natural state for most of us—we get exhausted and burnt out. When we are in a state of compassion—a state of being that takes practice and skill and intention—we remain resilient and energized.

In Dr. Singer's research, she demonstrates this with Buddhist monks who have trained in the practice of mindfulness—a skill of practicing compassion—for more than two decades. She shows them videos and pictures of people suffering while studying their brain activity. For the control group, she asked them to stay in a state of mindful compassion. This group was able to concentrate and view the pictures of suffering for many hours. When she asked the study group to shift into a place of empathy, they didn't last past 20 minutes before feeling exhausted and needing to take a break to reset.*

When I was a child, we received letters in the mail, and we were able to choose when we opened them, when we read them, and when we wanted to respond to them. If we wanted to watch the news, we could turn on the TV and choose to watch the news. We exposed ourselves to others' lives and the world on our own schedule, our own choosing.

Today, we are bombarded with hundreds of e-mails, tons of social media information, and thousands of images on a daily basis. The apps and programs on our computers interrupt our daily activities with notifications and sounds that give us adrenaline and dopamine pumps in the brain, which create a cortisol-based stress response. Dopamine—an addictive chemical in the brain—demands that we seek pleasure and satisfaction. We keep clicking, keep looking for that next article, that next text message, that next Instagram post that is going to help us feel better about our lives. That's a lot for the brain to handle. So when the natural reaction for our brains is a state of empathy, our brains are exhausted soon after picking up our phone or turning on the computer. As a species, we are all exhausted.

If you're wondering, "Dr. Milspaw, why are you even going into this?" It's because we're talking about retraining the brain out of pain, which requires trying to minimize the amount of stress and trauma we absorb

* This research is available on her website: https://taniasinger.de

from the world around us. When we practice mindfulness, we practice shifting our brains into a state of compassion. When we practice bilateral stimulation, we practice the "clean out" process our brains need to let go of the thousands of incoming data points of everyday life—especially the stressful ones. Remember, your brain is lighting up in the same way as the person you're paying attention to. Therefore, even if you've lived a stress-free life, your brain still needs help taking out the trash. **This mental clean-out process is necessary for optimal health and well-being. Mindfulness helps us do this.**

Am I saying that empathy is bad? Certainly not. Empathy gives us the ability to connect with each other. We're a social species; our brains need to connect. In fact, **if you grew up in a stressful household, your empathy response is probably really strong because it served as a survival skill.** In a stressful household, it becomes necessary to know the emotional status of your caretakers and parents. Commonly, children feel responsible for what's happening in their environment because they don't understand the adult world. Their *perspective,* which is developmentally appropriate, is that the world revolves around them. So if something is wrong, it must be their fault (in their mind).

Consequently, children absorb too much responsibility for managing everyone else's feelings in the home. If there's a lot of unmanaged emotion, children learn to manage others' emotions instead of managing their own. While empathy is a skill because it allows us to tune into what's happening in our environment, and specifically in regard to other people, empathy can cause our childhood "take-aways" to be self-blaming, shaming, and overwhelming. If you see your own childhood in this story, know that this experience causes a "wind-up" in the nervous system, paving the way for anxiety, depression, chronic pain, and illness.

Dr. Singer's research demonstrates that the skill and motivational drive to practice compassion is created by practicing awareness of others' suffering and being able to self-regulate and balance your emotional state. See the illustration on the next page.

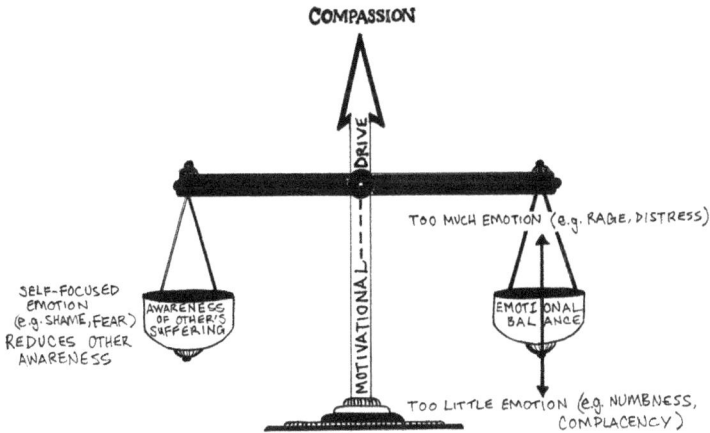

Mindfulness provides the skills you need to develop and strengthen your ability to experience and practice a compassionate presence with yourself and others. The practice of mindfulness trains these two skills via three different pathways: (1) presence, (2) perspective, and (3) affect. I list below these three different pathways and the specific mindfulness exercises that strengthen that skill:

1. Presence: Our ability to be attentive and interoceptive (attuned to our body's inner signals)
    a. Body scan
    b. Breathing exercises

2. Perspective: Our ability to zoom out and see things from other viewpoints
    a. Mindful journaling
    b. Observing our thoughts

3. Affect: Our ability to have an open heart, emotional acceptance, and positive regard for another person
    a. Loving-kindness meditation
    b. Heart-centered meditations

Can you think of one exercise that encourages you to do all of these practices at once? Meridian tapping! The process of EFT encourages you to tune into your physical sensations (presence), process your thoughts (perspective), and regulate your emotions (affect). Neverthe-less, I encourage the practice of all of the above, because, why not?*

Meditative Mindfulness

Meditative mindfulness is when we're closing our eyes, being still, and focusing the mind in a particular way. There's a variety of meditative mindfulness exercises, including guided visualizations, body scans, loving-kindness meditations, concentration-based meditations, and con-templation-based meditations. As you may remember from the pyramid process you drew near the beginning of this book, meditative mindful-ness is the top of the pyramid. We want to train our brains to visualize the healing outcome that we want to help guide and support the body in that direction.

As we learned from Tania Singer, mindfulness-based meditations help our brains practice the skill of compassion, which strengthens our re-silience and prevents burnout. We also see meditative mindfulness be extremely beneficial in our everyday lives, whether we realize it or not. We see the practice of visualization in sports psychology, virtual reali-ty, business performance trainings, and even flight school simulations. Visualizing has a profound effect on how your body is acting, how your body is feeling, and how your body is performing.

All meditations are for the purpose of getting you out of rumination—the repetitive and decentering, upsetting thought patterns. Rumination is defined as any thought that causes, maintains, or exacerbates the fight-or-flight response caused by the activation of the sympathetic nervous system. You want the opposite. You want the relaxation response. The relaxation response, in contrast to the deeply distressing nature of rumi-nation, is a state of mind and body where you feel deeply relaxed, where your physiological indicators (such as your vital signs) are within the range for a healthy, relaxed person. This is the state where your body is

---

* At the time of writing this chapter, Netflix had a series called *Headspace: A Guide to Meditation* composed of eight 20-minute episodes that each include 10 minutes of science and 10 minutes of a mindfulness exercise. It's a great introduction to mindful-ness and a variety of ways to practice mindfulness.

resting and healing, a state where you feel inner peace and your body feels well-being.

When you practice contemplative meditation, you can focus not only on inner or outer, subjective or objective experiences, but also on concepts, ideas, constructive thinking, emotionally fulfilling experiences, spiritual openings, etc. In other words, just about anything that is easily accessible, not unpleasant. Contemplative meditation can lead to peace, and what some call "alignment" and "centering," as it leads to a relaxed state. Because breath meditation is not guaranteed to get you into the "decentered" place, you should not make relaxation the goal, because if you make relaxation the goal and don't achieve it, you are likely to become upset and start to ruminate on whatever meaning you place on it (i.e., "See, I'm the world's worst meditator. I can't even do this right, therefore I'm no good"). Therefore, whatever your experience, just be with it and accept it.

Mindfulness-Based Cognitive Therapy (MBCT) is a descendant from standard Buddhist meditation practice, which is predominantly breath meditation and utilizing the breath as the main object of concentration and contemplation. However, experienced meditators from other meditative disciplines will tell you that other contemplative meditation practices, such as focusing on mantras and ideas, will also stop rumination and take you to that peaceful place. See Appendix B for more ideas on what you can use in your personal practice of contemplation meditation.

MBCT guides you to practice mindfulness in an effort to become aware of your thoughts more often so you have more opportunities to change those thoughts. Additionally, as discussed earlier, when you add mindfulness training to a Cognitive-Behavioral Therapy approach, you significantly decrease relapse rates because you're training your brain and healing your brain, rather than just trying to "think or do differently." MBCT supports all of the exercises we've explored so far in this book because it invites you into the present moment to observe what's going on, calm your system, and then decide what you want to do about it.

As you practice mindfulness, you're healing your brain. As you're healing your brain, you're able to reprogram your brain. As you reprogram your brain, you retrain your brain to respond differently to incoming stimuli. When you do this, you've mastered your nervous system and can heal your experience of pain.

Let's practice what you've learned. I recommend doing the following exercises in this particular order and all together for the most beneficial experience.

EXERCISE: QUICK I SPY

I'm going to guide you through the "Quick I Spy" mindfulness exercise. Then we're going to do a little bit of tapping, followed by some breathwork. Then I'm going to encourage you to move into a guided visualization. You can choose to listen to these links separately, or you can read the script below and allow your brain to enjoy the journey.

Before we begin, take a moment to think about where you want to go with the visualization. I'm going to ask you to remember a time when you felt most peaceful and relaxed. Take a moment to write down where you want to go. Maybe it's a place that you've been, maybe it's a place that you've imagined, or maybe it's your own personal sanctuary in your mind that you've created. Choose a place that helps you feel peaceful and relaxed. If it's a memory, this helps wake up the cellular memory and deepen the relaxation. Be sure to include the following details in preparation:

- Where are you?
- What do you see?
- What do you hear?
- What do you smell?
- What do you taste?
- What do you feel against your skin?
- Who are you with?
- What are you doing?

Now that you've prepared for the final visualization, let's start with the five senses. Take a moment to look around and notice what you see in your environment. If you're standing or sitting, make sure your legs are not crossed and your feet are planted on the ground, which can literally help ground you. Just like a copper wire grounds the outlets, your feet can help ground the electricity in your body by feeling the ground, and it helps calm the nervous system. When your arms are crossed or when your legs are crossed, this causes disturbances in your ANS. Even your primary care physician will probably ask you to uncross your legs before taking your blood pressure. Crossing the legs and arms over each other increases heart rate and blood pressure. Therefore, to really help calm things down, you want your body to be parallel.

OK, take a long inhalation and notice what you hear. What sounds do you hear in your environment?

Remember to breathe long inhalations, and allow long exhalations. Notice what you smell. What smells and aromas are in the air? Remember to breathe. Notice what tastes are in your mouth. What do you taste? As you exhale slow, steady exhalations, notice what do you feel against your skin? What is the temperature of air against your skin? Can you notice the sensation of your clothes, and the weight of your hair?

Great job! Now that you've checked in with all five senses, we've established a sense of safety in your environment, so now it feels safer for your brain to move inward. I invite you to imagine seeing something that easily brings a smile to your face. Breathe in. Breathe out. Imagine hearing something that easily brings a smile to your face. Breathe in. Breathe out. Imagine smelling something that easily brings a smile to your face. Breathe in. Breathe out. Imagine tasting something that easily brings a smile to your face. Breathe in. Breathe out. Imagine feeling something that easily brings a smile to your face.

Great job! As you now begin tapping on the side of the eye, set an intention to remember those five things that easily put a smile on your face, knowing that you can return to those five items at any time to help you smile, to help shift your mind's focus, your heart's focus, your body's focus.

Tapping Sequence to Release Fear of Pain

Now, tap on the side of your hand and begin noticing what remains in your awareness physically, mentally, emotionally, and spiritually. Follow the tapping points as you go through the following statements:

- Even though I feel this way, I choose to love and accept myself.
- Even though I'm aware of some of these sensations and emotions, I'm open to believing that I can feel better.
- Even though these thoughts, beliefs, and sensations have been there for a long time, I'm willing and ready to do my best to heal my mind and heal my body.
- I am here, after all, reading this book and practicing these exercises.
- Maybe I'm more ready than I think.
- I'm noticing how I feel.
- I'm noticing what's on my mind.
- I breathe in.
- I breathe out.
- I'm noticing the physical sensations and the emotions that those sensations evoke.
- I'm becoming the observer of my experience.
- I choose to observe with a compassionate lens.
- Even though it's sometimes hard for me to be nice to myself,
- I'm willing to try.
- It's hard for me to be aware of pain and not be upset about it.
- It's hard for me to be aware of pain and not be afraid of it.
- I recognize all of this fear.
- And I recognize where that fear comes from.
- I'm open to observing my body while releasing the fear.
- All this fear stuck in my body,
- All the worry and stress stuck in my body,
- I'm more aware of it now.
- I give my body permission to let go of what I no longer need.
- Even though I'm afraid this won't work,
- I choose to love and accept myself anyway.

- Just noticing the pain or the fear and the discomfort that may remain.
- Thank you, body, for trying to keep me safe.
- I'll take it from here.
- Even though I still feel this way, I choose to love and accept myself.
- I am ready to feel better.
- Even if I'm just going to do two minutes a day, five times a day, or five minutes a day twice a day.
- I allow whatever I'm doing to be enough.
- I'm ready to stop shaming myself and judging myself.
- It feels good to know that I can reprogram my brain.
- It feels good to know that I can calm my nervous system.
- It feels good to know that there are a lot of options on how my body can heal.
- It feels good to know that I'm not alone in this healing process.
- It feels good to allow my body to heal.
- It feels good to allow my body to heal.

Take a deep breath in—and release the breath with a long exhalation. Great job!

Heart-Centered Meditation

We're now going to move into a heart-centered meditation. Place both hands on your heart, bring your mind down into your heart, and breathe from your heart. Imagine being in the presence of someone who's easy to feel love for: a person, a pet, or maybe even a favorite place. Align yourself to imagine being in the presence of someone, something, or someplace that's easy to feel love for.

Notice the temperature of your heart space—the temperature of your chest. Is it becoming warmer as you allow yourself to tune into that love? Remembering that love has its own frequency, and it's a frequency that is very balanced, very harmonic, very soothing for the system. Allow your mind to float on the movement of the breath, knowing that distractions are normal. If you get distracted or something's asking that you focus on something else, that's OK. Simply notice what brought your attention away, and then bring it back to the movement of the breath. For now, bring your focus back into imagining being with someone who's easy to feel love for.

As you breathe in and as you breathe out, take 60 seconds to allow yourself to imagine being in the presence of someone, something, or someplace that's easy to feel love for. Noticing how good the warmth of the energy of love can feel inside your chest, as it helps warm your lungs, and warms your breath. On the next exhalation, allow yourself to change position or shift position to help you feel more comfortable as you move into the visualization.

Guided Visualization to Your Perfect Place

Allow me to guide you through this visualization. 🌳 *Note*: If you manage dissociative identity disorder or any other dissociative disorder, this exercise may feel safer for you if you read the script instead of listening to the MP3.

Allow your eyes to close and your body to begin to relax. Let go of anything that was on your mind, anything keeping you from being the person you wanted to be, doing the things you wanted to do, having the things you wanted to have; let go of anything that's been keeping you in bondage.

Over the next few minutes, listen to the sound of my voice, allowing all other sounds only to place you into a deeper state of relaxation. You know that when your mind and body become relaxed, you become more open to change, and when you become more open to change, your body and your life can more easily heal. Healing is a good thing. Pause and allow that thought to soak in.

I invite you to remember a time when you felt peaceful and relaxed. Allow that memory to come to mind now. As you allow yourself to remember that time when you felt peaceful and relaxed, in your mind's eye, in this memory, take a look around and remember what you saw in that place. Remember what you see now.

Notice how your hands feel as they rest in a relaxed position. Simply notice your hands, how they feel. As you remember that time when you felt most peaceful and relaxed, do you remember the sounds that you heard in that special place? Remember those sounds now. As you notice how your arms feel as they rest in a relaxed position, simply notice your arms where they are. Arms are relaxed, hands are relaxed, and your body is breathing all by itself.

As you remember that time when you felt most peaceful and relaxed, was anyone with you or were you alone? Remember that now. Notice how your feet feel as they rest in a relaxed position. Feet are relaxed, arms and hands are relaxed, and your body is breathing all by itself. As you remember that time when you felt most peaceful and relaxed, what was the weather like? Remember the temperature of the air against your skin. Remember that now as you notice how your legs feel as they rest in a relaxed position. Legs are relaxed, feet are relaxed, arms and hands are relaxed, and your body's breathing all by itself.

As you remember that time when you felt most peaceful and relaxed, what were the smells and aromas in that special space, that peaceful place? Remember those smells now. As you notice how the skin feels on your forehead and temples, allow the skin to release down, softening your eyes, allowing your tongue to rest on the bottom of your mouth, and your hair to hang on your scalp. As you breathe in, and as you breathe out, your face and head are relaxed, arms and hands are relaxed, legs and feet are relaxed, and your body's breathing all by itself.

As you remember that time when you felt most peaceful and relaxed, allow all the details to come to mind. Remember what made that place, in that moment, absolutely perfect? Remember that now.

Notice how good it feels to remember that time when you felt most peaceful and relaxed, allow the sensation of relaxation to feel like a warm blanket of relaxation as it flows over you from your toes all the way to the top of your head. As you breathe in and as you breathe out, know you can return to this place at any time in your mind. Notice how good it feels to be here. Take as much time as you need, begin wiggling your toes, wiggling your fingers. Begin coming back to today, back to now, back to this room. Begin hearing not only the sound of my voice, but all the sounds around you clearly and distinctly. When you're ready, taking a deep breath in and open your eyes, noticing how good you feel and how relaxed you are.

Now, as you rest in a relaxed state, say to yourself once more, "It feels good to allow my body to heal." Image that you have a magic mirror that you could use to see the future of your dreams. I want you to imagine looking into this mirror and seeing the life that awaits you as your brain, your body, and your life heal. First, notice how you feel in this future life. Notice what's around you in the life of your dreams, the life of healing, the life filled with love and vitality. Notice what's around you, and notice what sounds you're hearing. Do you imagine seeing the life of your dreams in this magic mirror? Notice who's with you and what you're doing. Good.

Every time you calm your nervous system, give yourself permission to return to this image, this future image, this image of where you're moving toward. Simply by allowing yourself to imagine it gets you closer to it. The power of visualization is the power of helping give your mind and body the blueprint of what you want. When you do that, in comes inspiration and ideas on what the right next step is for you. It starts with calming your system, and then it moves to visualizing what you want.

If any part of this meditation or visualization experience felt difficult for you, that's OK. This is where you're headed. This can be a good goal for you to work toward. Take one step at a time. Every day you're getting closer. Every moment you tune in and engage in the mindfulness practice of being in the moment with a compassionate presence, when you make that little course correction with your mind, you're more likely to stay there.

A SHORT STORY ABOUT MY PIANO

I used to have a really old piano that hadn't been tuned in a long time, and the piano tuner said, "Well, I can't tune it all the way today or the strings might break because they're old, but I can tune it a little bit today, and I can come back and tune a little bit next week. I'm going to have to come back every week or two for a few months, and then you can really get it tuned up."

That's what we're doing with your nervous system. When your nervous system has been in a place of fear, illness, and fight-or-flight mode for long time, it takes tiny tweaks of tuning on a regular basis to get you there.

Regardless, you're absolutely capable of getting there. I know that for a fact.

Chapter 9

Pain, Pleasure, and Relationships

It's all about connection.

This chapter is going to be talking about relationships* and how pain affects relationships: the relationships with friends, family, intimate or sexual partners, and most importantly, with yourself. With this chapter we're stepping into the spirit quadrant of the 4-D Wheel, the quadrant of connection and disconnection. How do pain and trauma affect your sense of connection and trust between your own mind and body? How does pain and trauma affect trust between you and your partner? Your friends? Your family? Your co-workers? Connection is in our tissues, in our nervous system, in our brain, and in our biofield. Where did you learn to love and be loved? Where did you learn what love means? Love is often paralleled with a sense of attachment, a sense of connection, a sense of feeling "magnetized" and drawn to someone. This can be felt as both a desire to be with someone—and sometimes a *need.* Connection, and our perception of it, is everything the universe is made of. In order to treat pain and trauma, we must heal our attachment-based traumas and strengthen our connections with ourselves and safe, secure people in our lives.

With your intimate partner, mental, emotional, *and* physical trust can be challenged, depending on how your partner responds or reacts when you're in pain. We call this "guilty by association." Even if they respond perfectly, beautifully, and lovingly all of the time, with the best patience in the world (which is hard for most people all of the time, but even if that was true) the experience of physical pain when your partner is

---

* For the purposes of this book, I am referring to a single partner. However, I am not, in any way, intending to ignore or dismiss the validity of polyamorous and polygamous relationships.

present affects trust on a neurological level because of how your brain chemistry changes when you're in pain.

Guilty by Association

When you're in pain and fear, that creates a distrust, even when you don't want it to. Whoever, or whatever, is around becomes guilty by association. The association can be connected with anyone or anything, including, but not limited to, a smell, sound, environment, or object. For example, the bedroom where sexual pain occurs, the dilator, the physical therapist, and, unfortunately, even the most trusted and loving partner. When I'm working with couples, assuming they've worked out all the relationship stuff (this is rare), they're saying, "I'm not sure why my body still tends to recoil when my partner sits next to me, comes in the room, or comes to give me a little bit of affection or intimacy. I can't seem to stop this reaction, and s/he takes it personally. There's a sense as if my body doesn't trust her/him. My heart trusts my partner, and my mind trusts her/him. I know I trust my partner, but there's a sense of pulling back."

When you look at the science behind Pavlov's dogs, where he observed dogs salivate at the sound of the dinner bell, you can understand the concept of behavioral conditioning. It can happen that way with relationships. If you're in pain and you've tried to have intimacy, affection, or sex and that leads to a physically and emotionally painful experience, the situation becomes guilty by association. After the association has been made, that partner's presence alone can trigger a pain response. This returns us to the concept of state-dependent memory and learning. The state that you're in and what's around you at that time is what your brain tends to click save. Unfortunately, your partner can be part of that trigger. This chapter is going to discuss how to change that. Using techniques you've already practiced, you can update your brain's software so your body can see your partner—and anything or anyone else—as safe.

EXERCISE: MIRROR THERAPY FOR CPP

Intention: Feeling comfortable with the self.

Begin your practice by engaging in intimate therapy on your own. Make it a point to take at least 10 minutes a day to be by yourself in a private, intimate space. Some women prefer to engage in this practice in the bathroom immediately after showering. When there, work with a hand mirror or other reflective surface to view your intimate areas. Take note of the anatomy of your vulva—the pubic mons, the outer and inner lips, the clitoris, the urethra, the vagina, and any pubic hair you might have. Pay attention to the aspects that make yourself uniquely you. Increase your familiarity with this part of yourself. When being present in this manner, engage in muscle exercises you might have reviewed prior, in session, or when at physical therapy. Mindfully push and pull the muscles in the area and notice how it feels as your body works. Be intentional in your actions as well as your thoughts. Consider the attractive parts of yourself. Praise your body for the many sensations it provides and the manner in which it functions. Find beautiful and unique things about your appearance. When you are kind to your body, it responds!

Also, have a conversation with your genitals. Talk to your body and all of its parts. Then pause and listen.

Your body always has the answer. Now take a moment to look at another part of your body with the mirror. Recognize the function, purpose, and beauty this part of your body provides. Feel gratitude for the health that exists in this part of your body. As you realize how all parts of your body are connected, look back at your genitals and invite the light of health to spread to that part of your body. Breathe in. Breathe out. Repeat.

The Science of Love, Attachment, Desire, and Trust

When looking at the science of love, attachment, desire, and trust, think about how you respond to *yourself* as well as how you respond to a partner. Research has been exploring brain maps and love maps for decades. John Money wrote the book *Lovemaps* in 1986, which explored the patterns of who we fall in love with and how that relates to the previous connections we've made in our lives. This was one of the foundational books for sexologists and psychologists in the study of brain maps and learned attachment styles. Sue Johnson has recently led the research on attachment styles and the neuroscience of attachment and brain mapping in her books *Hold Me Tight* and *Love Sense*. Hendrix and Hunt discuss the Imago Partner in their book *Getting the Love You Want* (I recommend the workbook version), which follows similar research on attachment theory.

We learn our foundational patterns of love, desire, and attachment in the first 10 years of life. Our upbringing and early relationship attachments program us for who to love and how to love. Early relationships teach us what a relationship should feel like and what trust looks like (not necessarily what it feels like). So what is trust? What is love? What is desire? What do you find attractive? What do you find arousing? What do you find pleasurable? What do you find exciting? Many of these answers are programmed into you as you grow up, whether you realize it (or like it) or not. It doesn't necessarily need to be Freud's Oedipus complex, but neuroscience demonstrates that he wasn't too far off the mark. It's more about an understanding of how the brain learns attachment. There's a great book by Ellen Galinsky called, *Mind in the Making*. She looks at the brain research of infants and children and how quickly children really learn what to expect, whether they feel safe in their environment, and when they are trusting the people to take care of them or not.

When we're looking at attachment theory, we're looking to answer the question, "How does the brain learn what to trust and what it needs?" For example, there are many decades where people were taught the "cry it out" method in parenting. Researchers at the time saw children as small adults and wanted them to become independent within the first few weeks of life. We're seeing the collateral damage of those good intentions. We see how neglecting to respond to an infant's cries creates trauma in the nervous system—a distrust of the environment and their caretakers. Babies left to cry learn that their needs may not be met, which amplifies the sensitivity of their nervous system. You see that in babies who are in the NICU for a prolonged period of time because they're not held as often as they're supposed to be. They learn to distrust their bodies and distrust that their needs are going to be met. NICU experiences can now be connected with an overactive nervous system, leading to a higher risk of anxiety, insecurity, depression, and chronic pain and illness. The good news is that our brains and nervous systems can be retrained and reprogrammed, for the most part.

Healing the nervous system, as discussed already, requires rebuilding trust between the mind and the body. Healing requires responding to the body's perceived needs and soothing the fears underlying them. **Fear-based learning can only be unlearned experientially**. Therefore, when your goal is to heal the relationship with yourself and your partner and anyone else, they have to be with you along your healing journey. We'll talk more about how to do that in just a moment. Remember: you need to be present in order to have a healing experience. You can learn what safe and secure feels like.

When talking about love, desire, and trust, what do those feel like? Let's return to drawing the body maps. When we explore and discover what emotions of attachment feel like, we can gain an idea of the sensations our body needs to experience **when trying to rebuild and strengthen connections.** Experience heals pain and trauma.

✏️▶ EXERCISE

Draw an outline of a body, like you did in Chapter 1. You're going draw what love, desire, and trust feel like physically. Start with love. Set a timer for 60 seconds. Close your eyes and imagine being with someone who's easy to love. As you imagine being with them, notice how your physical body creates various sensations. Bring your mind down into your body, and notice what sensations you feel as you allow the feeling of love to arise within you. After 60 seconds, open your eyes and draw the sensations. You can use diagrams and words. Here's mine:

Love

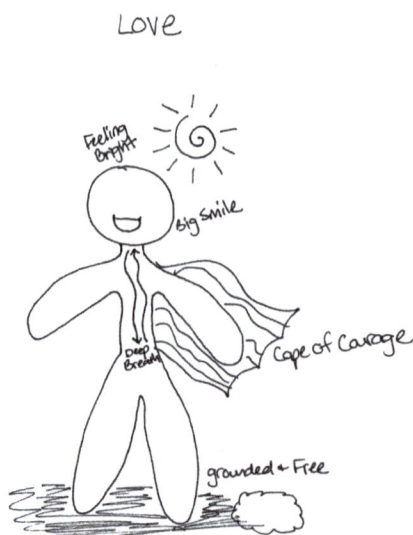

Now let's draw desire. Set a timer for 60 seconds. Close your eyes and remember a time when you desired something or someone. Desire comes in many different forms. Maybe you're desiring a cup of coffee, or a day to rest. Maybe you're desiring connection or soft touch. Notice what desiring—yearning—feels like for you. After 60 seconds, open your eyes and draw the sensations. Here's mine:

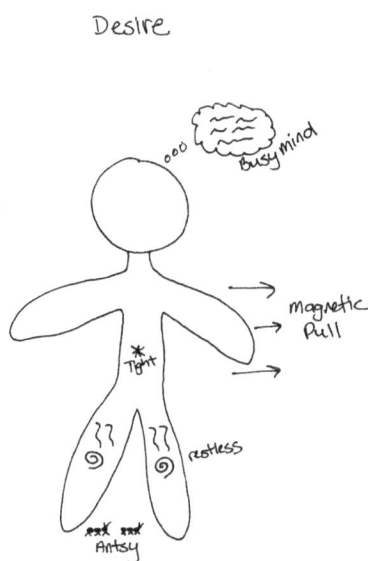

Desire

Now let's draw trust. Set a timer for 60 seconds. Close your eyes and remember a time when you trusted someone. Sometimes when I'm working with someone who has experienced trauma, they tell me they don't trust anything or anyone in the world. If that's true for you, then start with something small and basic. For example, you trust that gravity is going to keep you on the ground. Maybe you trust that the other driver is going stay in their lane when you're on the highway. Maybe you trust that your legs will move one after the other as you walk down the sidewalk. Those are some basic things you may trust. Maybe you've been privileged enough to have experienced deep trust with someone in your life. Maybe you've trusted a dog to protect you, or you've trusted that a friend would be there for you, or you trusted somebody with a secret they still hold for you today. Whatever feels most accessible and genuine for you today, remember a time when you felt trust. Tune into what that feels like for you. Even notice how your breath changes as you remember what trust feels like. Allow your mind to dwell on the feeling of trust for 60 seconds. After 60 seconds, open your eyes and draw the sensations. Here's mine:

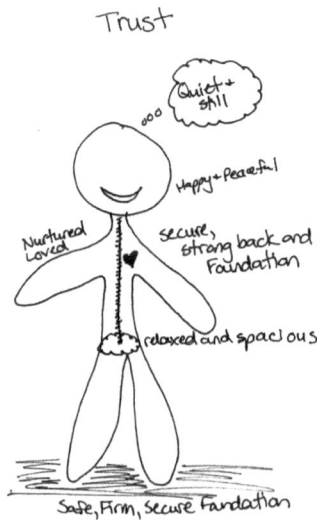

Trust

Quiet + still

Happy + Peaceful

Nurtured Loved

secure, strong back and Foundation

relaxed and spacious

Safe, Firm, Secure Foundation

Label these drawings in your notebook so you can return to them later.

Secure attachment mitigates the effects of trauma and pain. You can learn to create secure attachment. Secure attachment relationships reflect attunement, presence, safety, and consistent responsiveness. They include eye-gazing, affectionate touch, skin-to-skin contact, and initiating repair after conflict (85 percent more sustainable well-being in a relationship when you and your partner initiate repair). Who in your life represents secure attachment? Write down the names of these people in your notebook. They can serve as your anchors to helping your nervous system feel calm and safe, even when experiencing pain.

Draw, Show, and Tell

When you're having a hard time verbalizing or explaining what you're feeling emotionally, writing down how it feels physically can be a way to communicate. When you draw the physical experience, you tap into utilizing the same language and it can help get you to the same page. You may not know what it feels like to trust, but you know what it feels like to float on water, or feel your feet firmly on the ground, or feel your hands get tingly. Also, drawing your experience can feel very validating and provide an image for your brain to follow when you want to feel differently. Think about what it would be like to communicate with yourself, your partner, or a friend in this way. What would it be like to *show* them, instead of verbally telling them, what it feels like when they don't look at you, don't ask about your life, or don't respond when you tell them you're hurting. Often, when given a visual demonstration, it helps the other person respond more empathically, compassionately, and accurately.

On the other hand, when you get in your analytical mind (when you're in fight-or-flight mode) you get caught up on the content instead of the process. You talk from your perception and start verbalizing the narrative in your head, and you forget to zoom out, shift perspective, and explore the other layers of what's happening. In this mode, you're not able to get to the deep undercurrent of your emotions, and more importantly, fears. Furthermore, if you or your partner struggle to clarify or label what you're feeling, it can be really hard to know what to say. For example, if you're on the autism spectrum, or if you didn't learn how to talk about emotions growing up, which is very true for the majority of people, then you don't learn how to communicate your feelings in an appropriate or effective way. This can be a very frustrating and painful experience for everyone involved. When you can acknowledge that there is a mind-body connection and there is a physical reaction happening, describing what that feels like physically can help you and your partner feel heard, validated, and connected. It helps you get on the same page. Especially when the topic feels sensitive, such as when discussing painful sex, sometimes a drawing can speak a thousand words.

Pain and fear create a disconnection when what you need is connection. That's what your mind, body, heart, and spirit need. The neurochemical changes that happen are very different when you are either in a place of trust or when you're in a place of fear. The literature demonstrates that even if the physical pain sensation remains the same, our brains respond to it differently when we're in a place of trust versus when we're in a place of fear. When there's a sense of trust, even when your brain is receiving nociception from the nerves and muscles, the brain chemicals are different. This is a main reason for focusing on utilizing breathwork and bilateral stimulation to shift this fear response. When you're trusting, you can still experience a boost of oxytocin and dopamine with pleasurable sensations. Both of these neurochemicals tend to decrease pain and increase your brain's access to pleasure. However, when you're feeling pain and there's *fear* in your body, (i.e. there's fear of the pain getting worse, or fear of your partner making it worse, or fear of making your partner feel bad) this causes different neurochemicals to release, such as cortisol. Cortisol increases pain and decreases your brain's access to pleasure. Cortisol also increases nerve sensitivity and muscle tension. For pleasure and attachment, we must decrease fear and increase trust.

Attachment and trust are chemical responses learned experientially. The recipe for these experiences are taught to us. Some people grew up in a really quiet environment, and so quiet feels safe for them. Some people grew up in a very loud environment, and so that feels safe for them.

Pain + Trust =	Pain + Fear =
• Neurochemical changes in the brain ➔ attachment is created • Boost in oxytocin and dopamine • Calming of autonomic nervous system • Neuromuscular relaxation • Pleasure	• Broken trust • Neurochemical changes in the brain ➔ break in attachment • Cortisol spikes • Decreased testosterone • Upregulated nervous system • Muscle tension and spasms • Nerve sensitivity

When you have always had someone available and responsive, you learn this equals love. Some people learn the opposite. If their parent or caretake was not available and responsive, and not fulfilling their needs, then these people learn that is love because that is what feels *familiar*. **If it's familiar, it's safe to the brain. If it's unfamiliar, it's unsafe until proven otherwise.** The same thing goes with attachment styles. What was the attachment like with your parents or caretakers? What was the attachment like that you observed between your parent and their partner? Also, it's not only caretakers and parents who train our brain's attachment styles, but also siblings, teachers, and coaches. All of those relationships create and program your brain to what attachment styles you tend to have later on in adulthood.

In regard to pelvic and sexual pain, that part of the body refers to the lower chakras. The root and sacral chakras are all about that sense of trust, security, and safety. (See "Chakras Related to Pelvic and Sexual Pain" in Appendix D.) If you are navigating pelvic and sexual pain, it's worth exploring and strengthening your self-esteem, your sense of self, and your sense of security. Do you feel safe and secure at home? Do you feel safe and secure in your relationship? Is there a sense of walking on eggshells at work with your boss? There are many different ways that you relate and interact and connect or disconnect from other people in your life. It is worth your time to become aware of these patterns so you can start to address them and increase your access and opportunity to feeling safe and secure. The exercises in this book give you the resources you need to jumpstart that journey. When you feel safe and secure, your pelvic floor will relax. Guaranteed.

Attachment, Trauma, and Pain

Emily Nagoski does a great job of talking about the power of attachment styles and the importance of safe, trusting communication when building a healthy, pleasurable, and sustainable relationship. In her book, *Come As You Are*, she provides a chart, adapted here, that reviews the differences between the three basic attachment styles.

The best attachment style for a calm nervous system and relaxed pelvic floor is secure attachment. Secure attachments help us feel safe and relaxed. That's what calms the nervous system. That's what the pel-

Secure Attachment	Anxious Attachment	Avoidant Attachment
• It feels comfortable to share my private thoughts, feelings, and internal experiences with my partner. • I rarely worry about my partner choosing to leave the relationship. • I am very comfortable being close to my intimate partner. • It helps to turn to my intimate partner in times of need.	• I'm afraid I will lose my partner's love and affection. • I often worry that my partner will not want to stay in a relationship with me. • I often worry that my partner doesn't really love or care about me and my internal experiences. • I worry that intimate partners won't care about me as much as I care about them.	• I prefer not to show a partner how I truly think and feel. • I find it difficult to allow myself to depend on intimate partners. • I don't feel comfortable opening up to intimate partners. • I prefer not to be too close with intimate partners.

vic floor needs in order to be able to relax. You need to feel secure, safe (emotionally and physically), and trusting of the people and the environment around you, and you need to trust your body. Take a moment to think about what column you relate to the most. Please keep in mind: This is *not* about judging yourself or shaming yourself, because you learned these patterns growing up! There you are, as a child, "downloading" these paradigms of anxiety, avoidance, or security. We tend to be drawn toward both the positive and negative aspects of the caretakers we had while growing up. We're drawn to the positive aspects because those neural nets got connected with feeling loved. We're drawn to the negative aspects because we unconsciously seek to heal those wounds, so we end up reliving similar patterns we observed in an effort to create a different outcome.

When we find ourselves in a codependent relationship, we have an overabundance of *need* to experience the same emotion and share the same perspective. Did you grow up learning to feel responsible for how your parents felt?* As children, which I mentioned earlier in the book when discussing DIMs, we automatically feel responsible for the emotional well-being of our caretakers. However, if caretakers *confirm* this responsibility, that makes it more challenging to reprogram. For example, did you ever hear, "You made me feel that way," or, "You made me do that," or, "You made me react that way" ? As we reflect on our upbringing and our brain maps, the pieces of the puzzle start to come together. **Attachment styles are learned.** Explore this part of your life with compassionate curiosity. Ask yourself, "How did they teach me that? How did I learn that it wasn't safe to express my emotions? Who taught me that?" **Utilizing mindfulness as a way of being compassionately curious is the first step to healing and reprogramming our brains for healthier and more secure attachment styles.**

---

* I recommend the books *Codependent No More* by Melody Beattie and *Will I Ever Be Good Enough?* by Karyl McBride if you identify with either anxious or avoidant attachment styles.

EXERCISE

Take a moment to write down what breaks trust for you.

As you probably have already listed in your notebook, fear, pain, ego-centered listening, and judgement are some of the main experiences that can break trust in any relationship. The first is fear and pain. When you're in fight-or-flight mode due to pain and fear, trust becomes broken by accident in your relationship. How do you tend to respond to your partner and would you respond differently if you didn't have that fear? How do they respond to you? How do you respond to yourself? If you've been in a place of fight-or flight-mode or you've been in pain, particularly during intimate experiences, your partner's body really is going be guilty by association, and you will start to respond to them accordingly.

Ego-centered listening is when we're listening to rebut, listening to fix, listening to be right, and listening to defend. Much of this comes from the space of insecurity and anxious attachment. Ego-centered listening can come from the need to make things better, the need to be understood, and the need to be heard. That's an important need: to be understood. When it's not met, it throws you into fight-or-flight mode, and all of a sudden you're in your default mode network, replaying the narrative of your childhood and, commonly, acting accordingly. When you're in fight-or-flight mode, there's that sense of urgency, and you tend to interrupt and feel like your feelings are more important than your partner's. What's great about relationship therapy is being able to slow it down and take turns. I love using the 4-D Wheel with couples. I'll have each partner walk the Wheel, just like what you did in the beginning of this book, and slowly have the partner observe what is happening in the mind, body, heart, and spirit. When they're processing or experiencing or observing certain things, the partner often watches in amazement, learning about the many layers that they didn't know were there. The 4-D Wheel can also be a great way to slow down the communication and practice holding space for each other. How do you help yourself feel understood? How do you help your partner feel understood? I'll fast-forward to the answer: heart-centered and spirit-centered listening. This means prioritizing the emotion and the energy of what is being felt and communicated, rather than the content, and making the relationship a priority. Heart-centered listening allows us to intentionally make space for a different perspective. Mirroring, empathy, and validation are key in helping your partner feel heard and understood. Feeling understood is the opposite of feeling judged. More to come on these concepts in a moment.

Judgment, impatience, and invalidation can break trust. They can sound like, "You need to hurry up and figure this out," or, "Why haven't you healed yet?" I hear that from partners so many times. **That response is coming from their own sense of fear**. Partners often experience fear of not connecting, fear of not having sex again, fear of not experiencing connection. Why? Because in our society, sex is a doorway to something else—and we learn it's the only way in (no pun intended). Brain maps, pain maps, and love maps are learned and inherited. What did you learn? Did you learn that penetrative sex is the "end all, be all"? Did you learn that penetrative sex that leads to orgasm was the only way to connect? When you have an honest, nonjudgmental, compassionate conversation about sex and intimacy, you can begin discovering a deeper understanding of yourself and your partner when it comes to sex and intimacy.* What does sex mean to you? What does sex offer you? What does intimacy offer you? You're wanting what's on the other side of that door. There are multiple doors to connection and pleasure and intimacy. Just because CPP stops you from being able to connect in specific ways, you can still choose to figure out ways to get to the other side. Sometimes you just stop trying because trust has been broken. Many people stop trying to even access what's on the other side of the door due to fear, pain, and distrust with their communication and emotional habits.

---

* See page 223 for list of conversation starters.

Your brain changes with chronic pain and trauma. These brain changes cause you to be in fight-or-flight mode most of the time. Consequently, you become more defensive, which can create more critical responses. Stonewalling happens when you shut down and don't know how to return to a certain conversation because it feels too raw, too intense, too vulnerable. With these brain changes, you can hold grudges, even if that's not your normal personality. That's what contempt is all about. **As you heal your brain, and heal your relationships, all of these behavioral patterns tend to soften because you're providing an opportunity to be only in the moment rather than lost in the overlap between past traumas, the present, and fears of the future**.

When I'm working with one person or a partnership, I immediately start talking about the importance of healing the brain and nervous system. I tell them, "You must heal the brain first or otherwise this talk therapy thing isn't going be effective in the long term," because when you're in fight-or-flight mode you have a shorter fuse. You're more cranky. Have you ever been "hangry"? This is when someone gets cranky when they're hungry—caused by an abrupt drop in blood sugar, which spikes cortisol, setting off the alarms in the brain. This can become more severe with chronic pain and stress, due to the central sensitization of the nervous system. When you heal your brain, it's going to be easier to address some of these things that are commonly present in the relationship. As you practice mindfulness, especially if you practice mindfulness with your partner, you can increase awareness and intervene faster when you notice these patterns occurring. Mindfulness creates the ability to "pause" and recognize and communicate: "I'm feeling cranky now. Can we please hit the timeout button because this isn't going to go where we want it to go." If you don't practice being present, you won't be able to be present or communicate effectively the way you want to when you're feeling that way. Many people say, "I'm always in pain, so I'm afraid I'll always be cranky." Well, fear of not being able to change is one of the first things I recommend shifting. You can work on that now if you wish!

🌳 Listen to the tapping sequence for "releasing fear of inability to change" on my website.

John Gottman has decades of research demonstrating four main negative communication patterns that can break trust and attachment in a relationship, which he calls the "Four Horsemen." The Four Horsemen include defensiveness, contempt, stonewalling, and criticism. I recommend viewing a descriptive two-minute video on his website: www.gottman.com. In this video, he also describes the antidote to these four behavioral patterns.

When you train your system to shift out of fear, you can return to a place of trust. Researchers from the Neuro-Orthopaedic Institute of Australia observed people in the emergency room and rated their experiences of tissue damage and pain levels. They found that they did not always correlate.* As discussed earlier, fear and distrust change your perspective and your experience of things. Practice the exercises in this book to shift fear and insecurity, and practice mindfulness-based intimacy exercises to build trust and connection. When you do both of these things, you create your door to intimacy and pleasure.

Do not judge yourself if you recognize that you do any of these fear-based behaviors. Instead, recognize that these behaviors are often a side effect of your upbringing, along with the brain changes that pain and trauma create. As you're doing these exercises to heal yourself, you're doing what you need to do to be able to change your part in the relationship. Your accountability and willingness to make a change in-and-of-itself is *really* powerful. When you're looking at healing relationships, whether it be the relationship with yourself, between you and a partner, between you and friends or parents, or other people, think about how you create trust. Healing starts with initiating an intention and inviting an opportunity to repair—be it your body or your relationships.

Creating trust requires you to become more curious, more mindful. **Mindfulness transforms distress into curiosity**. You want to be able to notice you're feeling triggered so you can ask more questions. Don't ask "why" questions. **"Why" comes across as judgment. Instead, ask "what" or "how" questions.** For example, you might ask, "What just

---

* See Lorimer Moseley's brilliant book, *Painful Yarns* for *true* stories about pain told in an educational and humorous manner.

happened, I'm confused?" You're playing the confusion card. You're shining a spotlight on the mismatch of your intention and their perception. "I feel like what I said isn't matching your reaction. Can you please help me understand what happened just now?" If you're still rebuilding trust in a relationship, the need to slow it down and utilize communication charts (like the one in Appendix C) can be helpful to not only identify a behavior that your partner does that triggers you, but also what they can do to help you feel loved and cared for. Take a moment to explore these charts now. What are the behaviors that tend to trigger you? What do these behaviors make you feel? How do you tend to react? Recognizing that your reactions are coming from a fear can help slow down the assumptions. Finally, what do you want instead? As my first work manager would say, "If you come to me with a problem, you need to also bring me a solution." Of course, sometimes we don't always have one. But you don't have to figure this out alone. Work together with your relationship(s) to soothe your fears. **The more you begin to recognize and soothe the fear in yourself, the easier it will be to do so for your partner.**

EXERCISE

Take a moment to be curious. In your notebook, write down the fears that accelerate your reactions. You could fill in the statement, "I feel scared when I believe _____," or "I fear [insert belief] when you [insert behavior]." Next, think of at least one behavior your partner can do to show you love and care.

Here's a common example I hear: "I feel scared when you tell me you need and want more sex. I immediately feel not good enough, and I'm sad and I'm hurt, and then I withdraw because I'm afraid that you don't care." Often, if a partner hears this, it can trigger defensiveness. That sends you down a path of arguing about the fear, rather than soothing the fear. So while a normal defensiveness response sounds like this, "What do you mean I don't care? How dare you accuse me of not caring." A response of curiosity and care sounds like this, "I'm sorry you're feeling afraid of me not caring. I care about you deeply, and I don't want you in pain. The message I'm trying to send is that I miss touching you and want to be closer to you." When you think about this exchange—does it feel familiar? **What do you do to try to connect after a disconnecting moment? What do you need from your partner in that moment that would be helpful?**

Sometimes, people say to their partner who is desiring more affection, closeness, intimacy, "I feel like you're not taking my experience into consideration." In the meantime, the partner feels misunderstood because they were seeking only to share their desire of them. How does that tend to be perceived and interpreted within yourself? When you're perceiving or feeling those things, how are you reacting? Are you asking for clarification? Are you clarifying the intention? Too many of those of you reading this book have sex through the pain. You fake it to try to save connection, but that doesn't save it. It breaks it. Pushing through the pain breaks the connection between you and partner, as well as between you and your own body. Pretending is dishonest and unhelpful. What is the fear that holds you back from honest communication? Where did you learn that dishonesty was safer than the truth?

Nevertheless, here's what you do about it. First, you want to really get down to answering, "When I'm feeling triggered by my partner, what is the fear that they're poking?" You can explore this answer with tapping, journaling while listing to bilateral stimulation music, writing a letter that you may never send, or asking your best friend for their opinion. Once you identify the fear and calm the fear response, you can tune into your intuition about it. When you neutralize the fear, your partner doesn't necessarily need to change that behavior, because they could still act that way, say those things, or do those things, but it's no longer going to trigger fear. Instead, you might actually be able to hear it: hear their feelings, hear their desires more accurately, and choose what you want to do about it. As you turn down the volume of fear, you return to solution consciousness. You gain access to your frontal cortex, and you can communicate clearly, ask the clarifying questions you want answers to, and then make a decision about how you want to proceed.

The goal is to gain an understanding of all the pieces of the power struggle, or the "dance" that we all get into with our relationships. It's attachment theory—and the law of attraction—all mixed into one. *Getting the Love You Want: The Workbook* by Hendrix and Hunt provides the CliffsNotes of the research and walks you through a step-by-step process of healing your relationship. The authors guide couples to answer, "What's my greater vision for this relationship? What are my values? What do I want?" as well as, " What tends to make us argue with each other? What leads to us not trusting each other? Where does this come from and what do I need to fix it?" The authors come from a perspective called the "Imago partner." The Imago theory follows the brain research in attachment theory. In short, the research concludes that you learn attachment in infancy and childhood. Your childhood caretakers are who you tend to be drawn to. The Imago theory says you are drawn and attracted to someone who not only has the most important characteristics of the caretakers you had growing up, but they also tend to have the worst characteristics of your caretakers, because the intention is that the subconscious is intentionally seeking out to replay those same relationships to heal those childhood wounds. With this algorithm, the relationship provides an opportunity to heal some of the deeper childhood wounds. As you heal the deeper wounds and the beliefs planted by those early experiences, you recreate trust between your mind and body that was broken through the pains of your past relationships.

Relationships and the Garden of Your Mind

Research details the variables involved in creating trust, which include neurochemicals in the brain. When you think about what creates and strengthens trust for you, what might that be? Some of my clients answer this question with, "unconditional love, dialogue, patience, understanding, feeling listened to, and feeling heard." We know that childhood creates a large foundation of our brain maps and associated programming. Think about what this means for you and your partner. If your mind is a garden, and your genetic and ancestral history was the soil, and the beliefs you downloaded from your caretakers were the plants, what does your garden look like?

Did you learn that love was conditional or unconditional? Did someone close to you move away or pass away—and if so, did someone talk to you about it? Did parents or caretakers pay attention to you regularly or only if you were doing what they wanted you to do? Did they pay attention to you even when you were doing what you wanted to do? The filter of your perspective and how you understand the world is programmed at quite a young age. The more you can be aware of what those programs are, the better. Just like the garden of your mind, water the plants that you want to grow. Recognize the plants that you didn't plant. How do you want to remove the weeds and plants that don't serve your higher purpose and higher self? How do you want to plant the seeds of what you want?

Mirroring, Validation, and Empathy

Heart-centered and spirit-centered listening helps you feel heard, acknowledged, and valued. It focuses on the emotional and energetic experience of what's happening, rather than the content and fear-based narrative. The key to being able to help your partner (and all parts of yourself) feel heard is mirroring, empathy, and validation. You start with mirroring, which has two parts. The first part is repeating the words your partner used, because it helps them feel heard. You're literally "mirroring" their words back to them. The second part of mirroring is asking for clarification. You want to make sure that you're perceiving the message accurately before responding. This step takes patience and practice because you're slowing down the conversation, even if your ego wants to rebut. You also want to be sure they say what they mean. Many of us can say things incorrectly the first time, especially when we're in fight-or-flight. It's important to give our partners an opportunity have a second draft (and sometimes a third and a fourth—we're human). Clarifying allows you to respond accurately and appropriately. Commonly, power struggles happen because you didn't hear the whole thing. You got into fight-or-flight mode, your brain shut down, and you stopped listening right before the end, which was actually really important and could have changed your entire perspective. Mirror what you heard. Did you hear it correctly?

Validation sends the message that what is being received makes sense. It demonstrates that you can see the information from your partner's point of view and can accept that it has validity from your partner's perspective. *It does not mean that you agree.* Empathy provides connection. You're offering reflection of the feelings your partner is experiencing about the event or situation. Empathy offers to connect through recognition of their emotions and demonstrating an emotional reaction on your part.

EXAMPLE OF MIRRORING, VALIDATION, AND EMPATHY

Partner 1: "You never* help out around the house. You said you were gonna do the dishes, and you didn't do them. You never do the dishes! Blah, blah, blah."

Partner 2: "I hear that you're upset..."

Partner 1: "No, I'm angry!"

Partner 2: (mirroring and clarifying) "Okay, I hear that you're angry because I said I was gonna do the dishes, and I didn't do the dishes, and you feel like I'm unreliable; did I get that right?"

---

* When extreme words are used, like "never" or "always," that's a red flag that your partner is in fight-or-flight mode.

Partner 1: "Yes!" *(Or this is where the partner can provide their second draft** if they want to try to say it more kindly and accurately.)*

Partner 2: (validation) "I hear that you're angry that I didn't do the dishes when I said I would. I get that. (empathy) I can imagine how you would feel angry. I can completely understand why you would feel that way. I'm sorry I made you feel that way." ~ pause ~ "Let me know when you're ready to hear my perspective."

While the process of mirroring, validation, and empathy can feel very scripted, it allows each partner to step down and step back. It provides a moment of mindfulness because it signals to your partner that you're *trying*. You're demonstrating an intention to have the communication follow a different path than previous arguments. **This sends the message, "You matter to me." This is the message of trust and creates secure attachment**. Also, when you hear your words and your emotion acknowledged and mirrored back to you, it creates a relaxation response. Suddenly, more parts of the brain light up, and the brain becomes a better listener. Good communication is about slowing down and making sure you get it right before you respond and react. The literature, and my professional and personal experiences, demonstrate that when you slow down, and clarify what was said, *you are offering trust and demonstrating goodwill.* **The basis of trust and attachment is the deep-felt sense and being able to say, "I can rely on you. I can count on you. I know I matter to you."**

** Most of you reading this would never submit a first draft of anything that you wrote, but when you say something, your partner sometimes takes the first draft and "clicks save," and then won't allow you to rewrite or edit it. How many times have you wished you had the opportunity to edit what you said—especially if it was on social media?

EXERCISE

Write a list of what helps *you* create trust with someone.

Start Healing Your Relationship with a Vision!

Just like a business plan, creating a path toward healing your relationship starts with a vision. (I have a big vision of bridging the gap between the medical and the psychological world.) From that vision, you have the value statement and the mission statement. From that vision comes specific objectives. Then you get to the action steps. Folks often try to do it the other way around and start with action steps.

Certainly, those actions can be helpful, especially when they match your love languages.* The 5 Love Languages® are: quality time, acts of service, words of affirmation, physical touch, and gifts. You could be doing so many things for your partner, but if it's not in their love language it may not have the intended impact. If your partner can't see the connection between what you're doing and the shared goal, it's a hit and a miss. Write down what you want and what you value. When you combine your visions and focus on shared values, you co-create the desired experience and outcome.

Even if you're not in a partnership, all of these aspects are really important. Healing the relationship with yourself is necessary to do either before working on a relationship, or at the least, at the same time. A simple approach to begin creating your shared values and vision is to complete a chart, like the example on the next page.

There are three columns: yes, maybe, and no. The chemical of love and desire can get the best of us, which makes us agreeable. But we want to set healthy boundaries and expectations for ourselves before we're blinded by love. For example, maybe I'm agreeing to connect with someone, but they have something in the "no" column that I said was a deal breaker. So, why am I agreeing to meet with them? Is that coming

* "The 5 Love Languages®" is available at: www.5lovelanguages.com.

from a fear of being alone, a fear of not finding someone better, or a fear of all these things? The three columns are about setting boundaries and expectations for yourself. Again, this can be used not only to create your ideal partner, but also to create your ideal self. Who is your ideal self? How do you hold yourself accountable for your own actions and choices that lead you down your life path? The "maybe" column means you could take it or leave it. When creating a foundation of trust, clarifying shared values and vision is an important first step.

Creating the Vision of My Ideal Self/Partner

Yes	Maybe	No
Healthy	Sports fanatic	Unhealthy
Kind and loving	Likes boats	Racist, sexist, etc.
Compassionate	College educated	Abusive
Accountable for self-care		Lazy
Enjoys travel, adventure, and exposure to other cultures		

Here are four YouTube videos that are worth watching, all of which talk about various aspects of relationships:

- "How to connect with anyone" looks at how eye contact creates a sense of connection, even between two strangers
- "The anatomy of trust" by Brené Brown, PhD
- "How to sustain a strong sexual relationship" by Emily Nagoski
- Esther Perel has a variety of different Ted Talks

EXERCISE

Shift your fears of setting healthy boundaries. Starting with the side of your hand, and moving through the EFT points, say aloud:

- Even though I'm not sure how to set boundaries or to stick up for myself, I accept myself, and I'm open to learning.
- Even though I never learned to set boundaries, I still accept myself, and I'm willing to learn.
- Even though it's not comfortable for me to think about setting boundaries or to say what I want, I accept all of me, and maybe I can give it a try.
- I don't know how to set boundaries.
- I find it hard to stick up for myself.
- I learned that setting boundaries was selfish.
- I used to be shamed if I said what I wanted.
- If I set a boundary, they will be mad at me.
- I know I would feel uncomfortable having that conversation.
- I don't want to hurt their feelings.
- They wouldn't like it if I set boundaries.
- I feel like I'm controlling them by saying what I want.
- I'm afraid of their reaction to me speaking my mind.
- I'm not good at speaking my mind.
- I'm not good at asking for what I want.
- I'm scared to set boundaries.
- I'm scared about how they'll react.

- I'm scared about what they'll say to me.
- I don't feel like I can set boundaries.
- They won't like it.
- Setting boundaries will cause more problems.
- Setting boundaries will make my life more difficult.
- I'm so scared to set boundaries, but I also know I really need to.

Take a breath in and release. Remember, focus on lengthening your exhalations. If any of what was said feels like it has an intensity level of above a 5 on a 0-to-10 scale, you want to repeat the script. When it gets below a 5, you're ready to tap in what you want.

Starting with the side of the hand, say:

- I don't feel comfortable asking for what I want.
- I'm not sure I have the right to ask for what I want.
- But what if I could?
- Maybe this is something I could try.
- Find a small step where I could practice.
- I can find safe people to start with.
- I can get in touch with what I want.
- I can be excited to start this journey.
- I deserve to be heard.
- I can know what I want.
- I can start to ask for what I want.
- I can give them an option of meeting my needs.

- They can't meet my needs and desires if they don't know what they are.
- I choose to be open to setting boundaries and saying what I want.
- When I respect my feelings and ask for what I need,
- I'm showing myself respect.
- I'm honoring who I am.
- I know I want that.
- I really want that—to feel respected and to have my needs met.
- I'm open to allowing that.
- I'm open to giving that a chance.

Take a deep breath in and release. Notice how that second script felt for you. Ask yourself if you want to go through that again, or add in any more statements to help it feel more authentic to you.

When beginning your practice of setting boundaries, you can start small! Start by interacting with someone who has no emotional bond with you, such telling the restaurant server that you didn't get the meal that you ordered or telling the server that you want the mayonnaise on the side.

How are you at setting boundaries with complete strangers? Is it easier for you to set a boundary with a stranger or a partner? How are you with hair stylists? Do you tell them what you want? Are you honest when you tell them you're pleased with the cut?

I remember how hard it was for me to set boundaries with strangers. Growing up, I learned to always be "kind and courteous." As the daughter of a judge, I needed to always "put my best foot forward," which was translated in my mind to pleasing others, even if it meant lying. I knew

I crossed a good line in terms of my ability to set healthy boundaries when I got my hair highlighted and it was not the color I wanted. It took a few days, but eventually I bolstered the courage to call my stylist and say, "This isn't the color that I asked for. Can I come back for you to fix it?"

Of course, this being my first time, I offered to pay her for her extra time, which she declined (graciously). I remember her telling me when I went back, "Alex, tell me sooner next time! It's easy to change the color—it would've only taken an extra half hour." I'm someone who loves saving time, so of course that was the selling point for me. It's become easier and easier every time.

Ultimately, it comes down to your sense of worthiness and sense of deserving. **Write this in your notebook: "I'm allowed to want what I want."** In a relationship, if you don't verbalize what you want, it's not fair to your partner, or whoever it is, that you're now frustrated with them because they didn't give it to you. Follow three steps: (1) figure out what you want, (2) give yourself permission to express what you want, and (3) work together to create the best desired outcome.

One last rule: Don't **"yuk someone's yum."** I learned this at Widener University during my first course in human sexuality. You don't have to like what someone else likes, but you don't have to be rude about it. This is hard for me when my partner is eating clams. To me, they feel like a ball of chunky mucus in my mouth and just looking at them makes my face squirm in a distorted way. For the sake of respect, I've learned to smile and focus on feeling happy that he's enjoying his meal. As you're reviewing each other's values, vision, and desires, don't yuk their yum. A simple, "No thank you," will suffice.

Rebuilding Trust and Intimacy After Trauma

One of my favorite resources for building trust and intimacy after trauma is a one-hour audiobook by Peter Levine called *Sexual Healing*. In it, he explains how trauma and stress change the brain and how that breaks trust, even when you love and trust your partner. He provides guided exercises and other great ideas on how to rebuild trust. One of his exercises utilizes a Structural Therapy and Exposure Therapy approach because it provides a visual and kinesthetic demonstration of the internal experience. I used to love doing this with couples in my office. It's a mindfulness exercise and a boundary-setting exercise at the same time because you need to tune into how you're feeling and set a boundary when you notice your system reacting in a fear-based way.

EXERCISE: REBUILDING TRUST

Stand facing your partner, about 8 to 10 feet apart.

1. Maintain eye contact and use your hand to signal your partner to begin walking toward you *very* slowly. You're tuning in with yourself, having them slowly walk toward you.

2. When you feel your body start to tense, hold your hand up in the stop position.

3. Then your partner stops walking toward you, demonstrating trust by responding to your body language and your request to stop.

4. Then you practice bilateral stimulation, tapping, or breath work to calm your nervous system.

5. Once your nervous system feels calm, repeat steps 1 through 4.

6. When you're about 6 to 10 inches away from each other, reach out, hold hands and say, "Thank you for listening."

It's important to remember that "stopping" your partner from coming closer is not a personal attack. Your body is reacting to a fight-or-flight mode trigger most likely due to your partner being present during times of pain. When practicing this exercise, you're teaching your body that you're going to listen and respond. You're earning your body's trust, and so is your partner. It's demonstrating and training your partner to have patience and to trust the process, and for the two of you to trust each other. Eventually, when you're able to have your partner walk toward you and your body stays relaxed, then you do the exact same thing with more intimate, sensate-focused touch.

In the same way, you stand in front of a mirror and when you notice that you're being unkind or critical or judgmental, step back. You stand in a way to demonstrate that when you're in that mindset, when you're saying those unkind things to yourself, you're creating a disconnection. You're creating a distance between you and you. Then, when you speak words of love, acknowledgement, and appreciation, you move forward. Consequently, your brain is visually seeing you step farther away when you're unkind, and becoming closer when you're kind. You want to feel connected with yourself in order to create a stronger connection with your partner. The more you're connected with yourself, the easier it will be to allow your partner to love you. Sometimes when you do this movement exercise, it really helps you acknowledge how often you're creating a disconnect with yourself and with your partners.

Sensate-Focused Touch—a Necessity for CPP

Sensate-focused touch is exactly how it sounds—you're focused on the sensations as you touch each other in different ways, using different levels of pressure and different textures. Begin with setting boundaries of where you want to be touched and what places are off limits. When navigating CPP, start with clothes covering the genitals, including the breasts. You may want to have clothes covering any other part of the body that feels highly sensitive and painful to the touch. Clothes act as a visual boundary.

When beginning sensate-focused touch, start with extremities: hands, fingers, toes, arms, and legs. You're basically starting on the farthest part away from the painful areas, and then slowly moving closer. Similar to the Rebuilding Trust exercise on page 208, you stop touch and movement when you feel your nervous system tense. Calm the system, then continue. Do not move closer to the trigger areas without verbal permission from your partner, and sensory permission from your partner's body.

A calm system is an allowing system. All of the exercises listed in this chapter focus on becoming mindful of your body's response, saying "stop" when there's tension, calming the system, and then proceeding. This is a trauma-informed way to gently expose your body to safe touch and pleasure. **Whether you're building trust in a general way or trying to increase your body's reception to touch and intimacy, practicing these exercises with yourself can be very important to do first**.

EXERCISE: MINDFUL TOUCH

This exercise can be done anywhere on the bod y. If you're doing this exercise on a partner, ask for verbal consent before proceeding with this or any exercise involving touch.

Find an oil or lotion that smells good and feels good on your skin. This doesn't have to be anything special; many people use olive oil, coconut oil, or hand lotion. CBD-based lotions* and ointments can be helpful to decrease inflammation and pain.

Get comfortable. Focus your attention on one hand. Then, very slowly and mindfully, rub it with lotion or oil. Apply it to your fingertips, then to the rest of your fingers, then to the spaces between your

---

* I recommend Amy Stein's CBD brands, available at www.wellnessxnature.com.

fingers, then to your palm, and then to the back of your hand. Spend 15 to 20 seconds slowly and gently rubbing it in. Notice how each part of your hand feels as the liquid first touches it, then spreads across it, and then gets rubbed in. Now do the same for your other hand.

(Safeguarding your body requires self-regard and soft, wise, and compassionate self-care. Caring for your body supports its health, its healing, and its settling. A well-cared-for body tends to feel better.)

EXERCISE: NOW I'M AWARE OF... WITH A PARTNER OR FRIEND

Mindfulness-based stress reduction (MBSR) is the practice of being in the present moment without judgment and without trying to change anything. The purpose of this exercise is to practice being in the present moment with the help of a partner or friend. *MBSR techniques such as this one can help increase communication and intimacy in any relationship.* This exercise also helps instill awareness and a sense of acceptance for the present moment experience.

- Begin by sitting, standing, or lying next to your partner, facing opposite directions.

- Wrap your arm around your partner's as if you were hooking elbows together, so you are shoulder to shoulder and your arms can feel the movement of your partner's ribs as they breathe in and out.

- Notice each other's breathing pattern. Are you able to match each other's breathing? Is someone breathing slower or faster than the other?

  ◦ Note: *This is a common time in the exercise for giggling or laughing to occur. This is normal! Allow the laughter to come because it releases the uncomfortable feelings that often arise from doing something the brain sees as unfamiliar.* ☺

- Say out loud, "Now I'm aware of _____" and state what you are aware of in **this** moment. Perhaps it's something you see, hear, smell, taste, feel outside of your body (the sun shining on a leaf, or cars driving by) or inside of your body (noticing how your clothes feel against your skin, or a thought that just crossed your mind)

  ◦ Note: *This is the practice of mindfulness, so it is important to withhold judgment. Simply become the observer of your experience and listen to what your partner's observations are of his/her experience.* **You are not replying to their observation,** *only listening. For example, if someone says, "Now I'm aware of my headache," the partner simply goes on to state something they are aware of rather than saying,*

"I'm sorry you have a headache." The partner could say something like, "Now I'm aware that s/he has a headache."

- This back-and-forth practice can last anywhere from 5 to 15 minutes.

- After practice, face each other and discuss what this exercise was like for each of you.

- Practice this again in another environment or a different time of day to experience new observations.

- The next phase is to practice this facing each other. You may also practice this while *doing* something—bring in other senses. For example, you can put lotion on each other's hands in a mindful way while practicing the back-and-forth response of "Now I'm aware of ____."

There are many ways to practice this exercise. Be creative and have fun with it!

Here are some action steps that can be useful in rebuilding and strengthening connection and attachment in the brain:

- In-depth conversations (see the Conversation Starters on page 223) and order the game "We're Not Really Strangers" from Amazon)

- Eye-gazing (see a great video called "How to Connect with Anyone" on YouTube)

214 | **Pain, Pleasure, and Relationships**

- Sensate-focused touch (i.e., applying lotion with loving intention, showering together— anything that involves 100 percent focus on each other without the distraction of a TV show or phone). Set the scene: soften the lights, add soft music, and turn off phone/computer notifications. Explore using different textures and different types of touch. A favorite activity is using finger paint and painting each other's bodies. This activity brings various textures and playfulness, while also requiring an enjoyable shower afterward.

- Create a "menu" that you can use for these special times. Edit this individually to suit your desires and pleasures. Then you can "order" from each other's menus.

- Prioritize special time together on a weekly basis (see Emily Nagoski's Ted Talk on how to sustain sexual relationships, available on YouTube).

EXERCISE: EYE-GAZING WITH LOVE

For an example of the power behind eye-gazing, see "How To Connect With Anyone" on YouTube. I recommend watching this five-minute video prior to doing this exercise.

Time for this exercise: 2 minutes (can be longer if desired)

1. For one minute, send your partner looks of love. Making full eye contact, allow all the tenderness, passion, and affection you feel for your partner to pass through your eyes and into theirs. No words are spoken and no sounds intrude; only love is passed from eye to eye and spirit to spirit. Partner: allow yourself to receive their love, absorbing it without question, without doubt or fear.

2. After one minute, gently squeeze your partner's hand to let them know it's now their turn.

3. Now the partner sends their love in the same manner. Allow love to be freely given and freely received.

4. When this second minute has passed, you squeeze your partner's hand. Then both say, "Thank you" aloud.

Some pointers to help you with the eye gazing:

- This is a very powerful connecting exercise. You may find it a little uncomfortable, or even overwhelming at first. You might laugh or want to look away quickly. Persevere. Your nervousness will pass as your hearts open more and more to each other.

- Don't worry about counting out exactly one minute. Simply carry on with your loving look for as long as you comfortably can. At first, one minute may seem like a very long time, but as you progress through your practice, that will change.

- You may find it easier to focus on one of your partner's eyes rather than trying to look into both. Experiment to see what feels most comfortable for you.

At the end of your eye-gazing, read this aloud:

"Couples assume that the relationship itself will carry their commitment for them. They can fall into a trap of automatic behavior—taking each other for granted, allowing passion to die, losing interest in sex, forgetting kindness and respect. It is essential to keep commitment alive by renewing it again and again and re-creating it from a new perspective as you change over time."

There are two main aspects to sustaining a strong relationship, let alone a strong sexual relationship, and it's about having and healing that foundation of trust. The first aspect, which we've already discussed, is creating a foundation of trust and attachment, creating and strengthening the belief that your experience is important to your partner and vice versa. The second is prioritizing each other. Are you making time for your partner? How are you showing up in the relationship? How are you each demonstrating that making time for your partner is a priority?

Let's return to the food metaphor. If you're not hungry, are you choosing to no longer go out to eat with your partner? Or are you choosing to enjoy their company while they enjoy a meal? Have you ever joined them to enjoy their company, and then once they started eating you realized you were more hungry than you thought? *This is what intimacy can be like.*

The food metaphor really works when we're looking at intimacy and pleasure, especially when it's "been a while" due to pain, stress, and trauma. With sex and with intimacy, the brain can tend to be all or nothing. Because of the brain changes that happen, black-and-white thinking becomes the default mode. If you're not hungry, maybe you don't eat it all. If, for example, you've learned that if you say yes to a kiss or if you say yes to cuddling, that means you're also saying yes to sex, and sex hurts. Therefore, you say no to all those things because A + B = C.

To follow the food metaphor, if you've learned that eating steak makes you sick, you may not even want to go to a steakhouse for dinner. You'll *definitely* not want to go to a steakhouse if your partner forces you to eat steak, even when they know it makes you sick. (If this is happening, literally or figuratively, you need to evaluate the emotional and physical safety of your relationship.) Another example is a difference in appetite. If you want to go out to eat and your partner orders three courses—appetizers, meals, and desserts—do they force you to eat all three courses? Do you force yourself to eat just as much? Hopefully that's not the case. Hopefully, you eat what satisfies you, and your partner eats what satisfies them, and sometimes that can be the same thing.

That's what great sex and communication is all about. You need to learn what feels satisfying. You need to learn what you both enjoy and where the differences are. You need to explore what you want out of the experience. If sex is the doorway, or if intercourse or penetration is the doorway, where are you actually trying to get to? Similar to food's purpose being about pleasure and satisfying hunger, sex is usually about pleasure and satisfying a need for connection. **Pleasure and connection is possible without penetration.** Mainstream media zooms in on the "T" zone of the body. Pelvic and sexual pain invites, and often requires, you to zoom out and discover all of the ways your body can provide you with pleasure.

 EXERCISE

Let's practice a new way to communicate with your partner. You're going to create something called a Venn diagram. Draw two circles and cut them out so you can move them back and forth to get a feel for what the difference feels like. One circle represents you, and one circle represents your partner. First, place the circles in a way that corresponds with how you feel in your relationship right now. Then place the circles in a way that corresponds with how you want to feel in your relationship after you've done this healing work.

Look below to see what couples tend to draw when there have been years of chronic pain, maybe months and years of not having intimacy and not having sex because it leads to pain.

This is what the drawing can look like when partners are feeling disconnected.

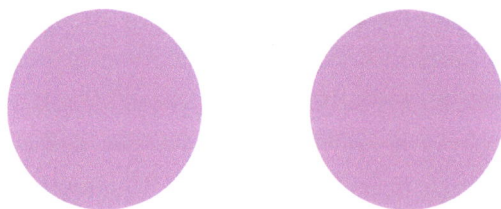

This is what the drawing can look like when partners are feeling trust and connection.

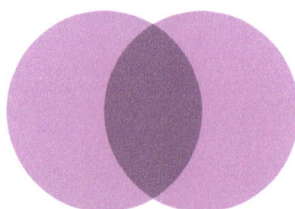

There are a myriad of ways the Venn diagram can look for each relationship, because different people want different things out of their intimate relationship. A picture is worth a thousand words. Drawing and using diagrams, such as this Venn diagram, can be really helpful at expressing what you want. It concretizes an abstract concept. When there's too much overlap, there's not enough to desire. Too much overlap leaves no room for autonomy or desire. The brain can't desire what it already has! Esther Perel explains this in her research, books, and Ted Talks. The brain really craves difference. Paula Abdul had it right: Opposites attract.

Talk About It

You want to appreciate your differences and acknowledge when it becomes difficult. How do you have conversations about that? Step one is communicating that you want to have a conversation. Step two is scheduling it and prioritizing it. This also gives both of you time to prepare and show up as your best self. When you take your partner by surprise and demand to talk about something, you aren't going to necessarily get their best self to show up for the conversation. Start with, "Can we have a conversation about our sex life Saturday after breakfast?" or "Can we create and talk about our intimacy menus this Friday after dinner?" Be specific about the day and time. As with any meeting, being specific not only increases the probability of it happening, but it demonstrates priority.

Overall, when we're looking at having pleasure and connection, relaxation is the doorway. Therefore, you must practice relaxing together. That's what Tantra is all about. Tantric exercises focus on eye contact, breath work, mindful presence, sensate-focused touch, setting intentions, expressing gratitude, and CONNECTING. You can also start with listening to a meditation together, lying outside and watching the clouds float by, or even sharing prayer and ceremony together. Shared experiences help us connect.

Instead of connection, mainstream media trains us to focus on physical arousal responses, including erections and vaginal lubrication. Meanwhile, physical arousal responses are different for men and women, especially when pain and trauma are involved. It's important to talk about this difference, because your experiences are different, and your brain's programming is different. These differences create an inaccurate perception of what's happening for your partner. Physical response does not dictate the emotional and mental experience of your partner. You have most likely learned to connect those variables. You may say to yourself, "If he doesn't get an erection, that must mean he's not attracted to me" or "If she isn't lubricated or if her vagina isn't allowing me to enter her, then she must not want to connect with me." You tend to really personalize things. "Thanks, mass media" (sarcasm here).

Instead of jumping to conclusions, especially if those conclusions feel self-deprecating or judgmental toward your partner, have a conversation. You can start with these statements: "I feel turned on when ____" or "I feel turned off when ____" or even better, "I turn myself on/off when ____."

The biggest sex organ is your brain, and being able to communicate about what your experience is can really help both of you understand each other better. You may even walk away understanding yourself better. What are the conclusions and the assumptions that you're making? You can build trust by saying, "Hey I'm making this assumption, and I'm reacting to it, but I'm realizing that this is the narrative in my head, and I actually haven't checked in with you about it." Talk about it and remember to practice mirroring, validation, and empathy.

Setting the Scene—Tips and Tricks

Creating the ideal environment and having some different props at the ready can be really useful. Here are some quick tips, tricks, and recommended supplies.

- Set the scene and consider all five senses. Choose the lights, the sounds, the smells, the texture of the sheets, and the tastes involved (brush teeth, have delicious drinks and snacks to change the palate, and enjoy on each other's bodies).

- Coconut oil, hypoallergenic lotion, and lube.
  - Slippery Stuff lube has been a top recommendation by pelvic floor physical therapists over the past 15 years.
  - I also recommend a CBD-based lube by Amy Stein (a well-known, kick-ass pelvic floor physical therapist in New York City) that works really well to increase circulation and to calm down nerve sensitivity.
- Vibrating massage balls by Pure Romance are really useful for releasing muscle tension and distracting the mind. Fun fact: The higher up the spinal cord is stimulated, that's what the brain focuses on first. This is why tapping your foot helps when you have to pee. The nerves from the bladder go into the lower sacral spine, while the nerves from the toes enter into the spine a little higher up. I have heard from many clients that using a vibrator on their clitoris or lower abdomen has eliminated pain from the opening of the vagina and allowed painless intercourse. You can play around with that.
- The Ohnut is a really great device to limit depth of penetration. This is a prop that you put on the penis to act as a "bumper" and also helps with peace of mind because you know the penis won't "slip" in deeper than you want it to go. It also doubles as a penis ring and provides pressure around the base of the penis, which can aid in erectile dysfunction. If you're a male with pelvic and sexual pain, and erections don't come easily or you lose the erection, a penis ring can be really helpful in increasing circulation in the penis. **When the pelvic floor muscles are tight, it decreases circulation, which is going to decrease the arousal response for both men and women.** For females, you can practice using the Ohnut with a dilator first to get a feel for how it works. When the deeper pelvic floor muscles are still really sensitive, especially that internal obturator muscle, a graduated exposure approach to penetration is very useful. The Ohnut comes in four different layers that come apart. As penetrative sex becomes easier and less painful, you can take one layer off at a time to allow for deeper penetration.

In summary, these exercises guide you to work together to:

- Become familiar with your anatomy and physical response
- Learn your physical boundaries
- Relax together
- Notice your body's response to different types of touch
- Create trust emotionally and physically
- Create connection
- Create pleasure

One of my favorite sensate-focus exercises is using finger paint on each other's bodies, because that can be a way that you can have fun. You're focused on the colors, the drawing, and the designs, but you end up just feeling different sensations. It can feel fun and creative, and it gets you back into touching each other in a way that feels safe, with clear boundaries being set. Then if that goes well, you can always take a shower together. Doesn't that sound like fun?

Think of foreplay as an attitude, not a behavior. Foreplay is everything we engage in between sexual encounters. Sometimes we forget about everyday touch and emotional connection. We often define intimacy as only what's happening in the bedroom, but cultivating touch outside of the bedroom can help keep those sparks alive. Foreplay begins the minute the last sexual interaction ends. We often think of foreplay as what we do to warm us up for sex right before sex, but we need the positive connections in between to help grow and foster desire. Real foreplay is the emotional, mental, and non-sexual physical connections we maintain in between sexual encounters. It's the energy and spark between us. Here are a few examples of foreplay:

- When you do the dishes and it's not your turn
- When you compliment your partner
- When you take the time to talk to each other after a stressful day
- When you order in and do a "date night" at home
- Non-sexual touch
- Rubbing the back of the neck
- Playing with hair

- Holding hands
- Kissing
- Cuddling

These touches outside of sex are setting the positive stage for your next sexual encounter. When you shift your perspective on foreplay, it becomes an attitude of consistently fostering connection with your partner rather than 20 minutes of making out and touch before sexual initiation.

What's one of your favorite non-sexual ways to connect?

More NLP* exercises that can be useful in relationship healing include:

- Mending a broken heart—a "movie theatre" technique that helps the brain neutralize painful moments in your past or current relationship
- Chords of connection—helps you heal your sense of connection with your partner
- Inserting resources—helps your brain access what you want to feel when practicing intimacy and sensuality
- Brainspotting—neutralize images that connect intimacy with pain and fear
- Creating a collage in your mind of images that remind you of sensuality

Conversation Starters for Sexual Health and Intimacy

- What is sex and what does sex mean to you?
- When you think of sex, what comes to mind? (Jot down any words, images, and associations.)
- How do you turn yourself on?
- How do you turn yourself off?

---

* Neuro-Linguistic Programming (NLP) is a set of techniques that utilize specific language to change the way your brain perceives incoming signals from your physical body, environment, thoughts, and emotions. More information can be found on the website of the National Federation of Neuro-Linguistic Programming: www.nfnlp.com.

- When do you feel most free in your relationship?
- Is there something sexual you long for?
- What's the purpose of sex for you?
- What do you wish you could experience with sex?
- What's the difference between sex and intimacy?
- When do you feel most attractive?
- When do you feel most tense with sex?
- When do you feel most tense with intimacy?
- What's the best compliment you like to receive?
- How comfortably are you with nudity?
- What sense (sight, sound, taste, smell, touch) do you enjoy the most?
- What sense do you enjoy the least?
- What sense feels most sensitive for you?
- What is a fantasy you tend to return to in your mind?
- What did you learn about sex and intimacy growing up?
- What did you learn about masturbation growing up?
- Was sex talked about openly in your family when you were growing up?
- Did you observe intimacy and/or affection in your family when you were growing up?
- Where did you learn about sex?
- What were the messages about boys/men, girls/women, transgender in your family?
- What are your favorite ways to be touched?
- Where are your favorite places to be touched?
- What are the rules in your sex life?
- Do you ever pretend? If yes, what propels you to pretend?
- What are your fears around sex?
- What are your fears around intimacy?
- What do you love most about your body?
- What do you dislike the most about your body?
- Do you ever wish you were more sexual?
- Do you ever wish you were less sexual?

- Do you watch porn? If so, what do you like about it? What do you hate about it?
- Do you need intimacy in sex?
- How has age changed your sexuality?
- What do you crave the most in your intimate life? Your sexual life?
- What props (if any) do you use in sex? Do you enjoy them?
- How comfortable are you in communicating your boundaries with sexual partners?
- Have you ever been loved the way you wish to be loved?
- Has anyone ever touched you or asked you to touch them in a way you didn't like?
- What metaphor best describes your sexuality?
- What object represents what you wish you could change about your sexuality?
- What object represents what you wish you could invite into your sexual life?

PLANTING SEEDS OF LOVE

Thank you for...	*Something I love about you is...*
It means a lot to me when you...	*One of my favorite memories with you is...*
When I think about you... (insert action) *It makes me smile.*	*When you...* (insert action) *I feel loved.*
I know you love me when you ...	*I have so much fun when we...*
I want to do...with you more often.	*I like that we work together ...*

...Wouldn't be the same without you

I see that you are struggling with...

[blank]

I am here for you.

Thank you for being part of teaching me...

I can tell it matters to you...

It helped me understand when you told me about...

I see your joy when...

I like the way...

I find it beautiful that you...

I learn about...

[blank]

From being with you.

I appreciate that you forgave me...

I enjoy...

[blank]

...together.

I think about you when...

I think your passion about....

Is beautiful.

I hope we can work out our

differences about...

I admire...

It means a lot to me when you...

I like that we are different about...

One of my favorite memories

with you is...

....wouldn't be the same without you.

I think about you when...

Use these spaces to write your own ideas.

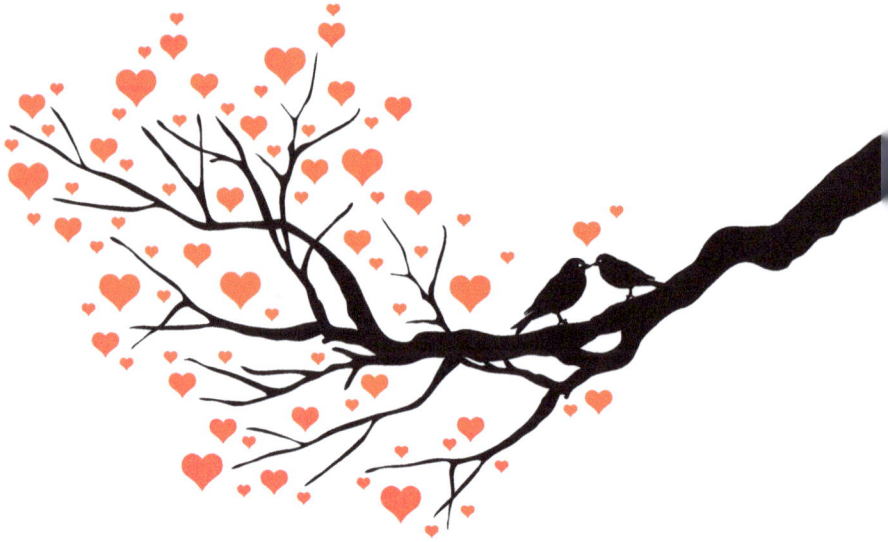

4D

loving intentionally

MENU ITEMS

entrees

- ♡ Manual play
- ♡ Masturbate together
- ♡ Oral sex
- ♡ Penetrative sex
- ♡ Role playing
- ♡ Using props/toys to increase arousal and stimulation
- ♡ New positions I'd like to try: _____
- ♡ _____
- ♡ _____
- ♡ _____

. . . .

desserts

- ♡ 5 minutes of cuddle time
- ♡ Shower/bath together and wash each other
- ♡ Lotion each other
- ♡ Meditate together
- ♡ Share a tasty snack
- ♡ _____
- ♡ _____
- ♡ _____

4Directions Counseling
Mind. Body. Heart. Spirit.

appetiz

♡ Compliment my appearance
♡ Say "Thank you" for something "I'm expected to do"
♡ Hold my hand
♡ Kiss me longer
♡ Run fingers through my hair
♡ Choose a date activity that you know I like, even if it's not your first choice
♡ Kissing my neck
♡ When you schedule me into your schedule – when you make time for me
♡ When you want to try something new with me
♡ 2-5-minute game: 2-5 minutes for me, 2-5 minutes for you, repeat
♡ Initiating "Planting seeds of love" card activity – 1 card each
♡ Acknowledge the sacrifices I make for our family/relationship
♡ Respect/honor shared space, especially after one partner just cleaned/tidied
♡ When I give you feedback, you say, "I'll try" instead of getting defensive/offensive

> i.e. "Will you please try to remember to put that away when you're done" –
> "Yes, I'll try. Thanks for letting me know that bothers you."

♡ Tone of voice. When you have a mindful, friendly tone in your voice that says "I love you. I care about you. You're important to me."
♡ Being playful - Initiate having fun, laughing, playing, with me.
♡ Reading scenes from Erotic/romantic novels to each other
♡ Shower/bath together
♡ Massage   o Feet   o Back   o Head
            o Hands   o Neck   o Full-body
♡ Sharing a healthy meal
♡ Eye-gazing for 4 minutes
♡ Harmonized breathing
♡ Completing Extragenital Matrix together (See page 234.)
♡ Creating "traffic" zones map of your body

> (red = don't touch, yellow= go slowly/be   gentle, green = YES, definitely touch)

♡ Discuss how you want to give/receive feedback during sex

> (i.e. tell me what to do, rather than what not to do; use gentle, loving voice; be encouraging; try not to make me feel bad for not getting it right the first time..or the second)

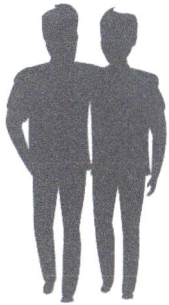

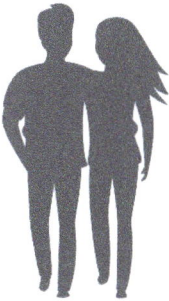

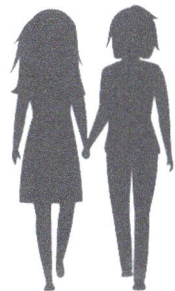

♡   Dance
♡   Play music together
♡   Spoon/snuggle
♡   Whisper sweet intentions/words of love
♡   Clean
♡   Brush hair
♡   Make art together
♡   Play outside
♡   Exercise together
♡   Yoga together
♡   Play a game
♡   Watch a funny movie
♡   Watch a sexy movie
♡   Share a fantasy
♡   Share: "You turn me on when…"
♡   Share: "I feel loved when you.."
♡   Share: "I feel desirable when you…"
♡   Share: "I feel appreciated when you…"
♡   Share: "I feel special when you…"
♡   Extra long cuddle
♡   Share/discuss one of your life's dreams
♡   Tell a story of one of your favorite moments you've
      shared with your partner
♡   Tell a story of one of your favorite moments in life
♡   Set the mood
      light candles, play music, prep the space for easy-to-
      access props and toys (lube, condoms, eye mask, lotion,
      vibrator, pillows, fruit, water, tasty treats, etc)

♡_____
♡_____
♡_____

Extragenital Matrix: Areas of Body and Kinds of Stimulation

	Hand stroke	Hand pinch	Hand slap	Lips suck	Lips blow cold	Lips blow warm
Hair						
Face						
Eyes						
Nose						
Lips						
Tongue						
Ears						
Lobes						
Neck						
Throat						
Shoulder						
Breasts						
Nipples						
Armpits						
Upper arms						
Behind elbows						
Lower arms						
Wrists						
Hands						
Fingers						
Sternum						
Stomach						
Abdomen						
Upper back						
Lower back						
Coccyx						
Buttocks						
Mons						
Clitoris						
Outer lips						
Inner lips						
Urethra						
Perineum						
Introitus						
Vagina						
G spot						
Anus						
Outer thighs						
Inner thighs						
Behind knees						
Calves						
Ankles						
Feet						
Toes						
Whole body						
Other						

©Gina Ogden, PhD, LMFT: *Women Who Love Sex: Ordinary Women Describe Their Paths to Pleasure, Intimacy, and Ecstasy*

Tongue lick	Tongue flutter	Teeth	Hair	Feet	Genitals	Other	Toys

Progressive Monthly Program for Partnerships Navigating CPP

This introductory program is for female pelvic pain clients in hetero-sexual relationships. The same guidance can be adapted for male pelvic pain clients, as well as for all relationship orientations. The most important part of this program is the inclusion of compassion, curiosity, and patience. We strongly encourage placing penetrative sex on the back burner until you have reached Week 5. This allows both partners to engage in these exercises without the pressure of performance. This is necessary when inviting the body to build trust and intimacy with the self as well as with a partner.

Remember that the program as presented below is recommended to take place at your own pace. Allow at least one week for each phase of the program, and do not hesitate to take longer as needed. Be patient and intentional with your body: These practices take time, and progress may not occur immediately. It is better to go slowly than to rush progress, which could set your pace back even further.

If at any time you feel pain or discomfort when conducting the exercises below, immediately stop what you are doing and remain still. Practice self-regulating exercises, such as mindful breathing or EFT (bilateral tapping), until the negative sensations you are feeling have ceased. Then you may continue as before or end your practice for the moment.

Month 1

Intention: Feeling comfortable with the self.

Begin your practice by engaging in intimate therapy on your own. Make it a point to take at least 10 minutes a day to yourself in a private, intimate space. Use a hand mirror or other reflective surface to view your intimate areas. Take note of the anatomy of your vulva—the mons, the outer and inner lips, the clitoris, the urethra, the vagina, and any pubic hair you might have. Pay attention to the aspects that make yourself uniquely you. Increase your familiarity with this part of yourself.

When being present in this manner, engage in muscle exercises you might have reviewed prior, in session, or when at physical therapy. Mindfully push and pull the muscles in the area and notice how it feels as your body works.

Be intentional in your actions as well as your thoughts. Consider the attractive parts of yourself. Praise your body for the many sensations it provides and the manner in which it functions. Find beautiful and unique things about your appearance. When you are kind to your body, it responds!

Also—have a conversation with your genitals.

Month 2

Intention: Increasing safety and comfort with the self while the partner is present.

Continue your practice from the week prior. This time, when you feel comfortable, invite your partner into this space to engage in this intimacy with you. Continue to be intentional in your actions and observations. Touch and explore the space with a gentle hand. Provide positive feedback, observations, and affirmations about your body, and encourage your partner to do the same. If you feel comfortable, touch and explore the area and continue to provide feedback and affirmations.

If you feel comfortable, invite your partner to do the same—place your hand over that of your partner's, and guide it over your anatomy.

If you begin to experience pain or aches, do not worry. Stop what you are doing and remain there and practice the breathing exercises you have learned until the uncomfortable feelings subside. This is your fight-or-flight response, and it is natural. Thank your body for working to keep you safe, and encourage your body to know you are safe and well taken care of in the present moment.

Month 3

Intention: Increasing safety and comfort "opening up."

Continue to embrace the practice as you have been doing over these past few weeks. This week, when you are ready, begin to incorporate utilizing a dilator* or your fingers, as guided by your pelvic floor physical therapist. Practice these actions on your own at first before inviting your partner to do this with you. Your partner can observe how you approach, explore, and eventually enter your body to learn what feels safe and comfortable for you.

Never force entry of anything into your body until you feel ready emotionally, mentally, and physically. This month, focus only on becoming comfortable with the use of dilators and fingers around the genitals. This creates a safe association between these objects and your brain.

Remember to be mindful in your practice and continue to offer yourself affirmations and praise for embarking on your healing journey. Notice the sensations that are encouraged from your practice. Notice how this part of your body offers you the capacity to feel such positive, sensitive sensations.

When you feel ready for it, ask your partner to join you on this part of your journey. Engage in mindful communication with your partner, speaking back and forth about feelings, actions, and observations in the present moment. Use "Now I'm aware of…" language, which you have previously discussed in session. For example, you might say, "Now I'm aware of a pleasurable sensation when I stroke my inner lips." Your partner might respond, "Now I'm aware that you are experiencing pleasure from stroking your inner lips."

Month 4

Intention: Increasing safety and comfort "opening up" with your partner.

Build on your practice from the past weeks by inviting your partner, when you are ready, to engage in the dilator and digital work with

---

* I recommend the dilator set from Pure Romance and Soul Source.

you. Begin the week by focusing on the outer portions of your vulva. Move slowly and intentionally, continuing to affirm and noting any observations using mindful communication. Continue to utilize mindful relaxation exercises. When either you or your partner notice muscles tension, or tension in general, stop the practice in place and engage in relaxation and mindful breathing. When muscles relax, continue the practice. Repeat as necessary. Your muscles tense to protect you. React to them with patience and peacefulness, and this tension will begin to subside. Notice this experience and pay attention to it. Ask yourself, "How do I intentionally relax?" Notice what works for you. During this practice, communicate with your partner. There is no such thing as too much communication. Ask and grant permission even for small acts.

Month 5

Intention: Playful Outercourse → Intercourse

Continue your practice, and be mindful and notice how the experience has been over the last few weeks. At this time, allow your partner to increase their physical engagement with you. Your partner has been welcomed into participating in intimate digital and dilator work with you.

As you feel comfortable, encourage your partner to bring their anatomy into this practice, as well. Your partner may begin by rubbing their genitals on yours. Remember there is no pressure to engage in intercourse or penetration at this point. Take the practice at your own pace. It is important to stop and practice relaxation exercises if there is pain or discomfort in order to continue to retrain the body. Remember to take this practice at your pace and to be assertive with your boundaries to your partner. Your partner loves you and does not wish to hurt you, so remember to communicate the feelings and sensations you are experiencing. As you feel comfortable, you may wish to encourage slow penetration, again going at your own, self-set pace. Perhaps your partner can begin with slow penetration, with just the tip. Remember there are no fast movements and no back or forth. When you are ready, let some small part in and notice how it feels. Continue to practice relaxation and communicate as necessary. Continue the practice and incorporate more acts as you are comfortable.

Beyond

Continue the practice as you find necessary. It may be beneficial to incorporate at least some time each day to be present and mindful with your body. Don't be afraid to move backward and forward between the steps incorporated above; the suggestions for time are just that—suggestions. Listen to your body and the signals it is sending you. It is OK to take time on this practice. You have so much time to get to know your body intimately.

Remember to allow your body patience as you acclimate to your new way of being present with your body and your partner's body.

Recommended Reading: *28 Days to Ecstasy* by Copeland and Link. This book provides a 28-day process that is grounded in mindfulness-based exercises intended to increase a sense of emotional, mental, physical, and spiritual connection. While you may want to change some of the language to fit your personal belief systems, the techniques in the book can be highly effective at calming the nervous system and increasing trust between sexual partners.

Chapter 10

Sound Therapy, Light Therapy, and So Much More!

As discussed in Chapter 6, frequencies are the hardware of our universe. In this chapter, we're going to talk about the healing frequencies of sound and light. Before we get started, let's practice two exercises that can help prime the brain for learning.

EXERCISE: STANDING MEDITATION

Allow yourself to stand with your feet hip-distance apart. For hip alignment, you want your toes pointing forward. Stand so your feet are underneath your sit bones, underneath your hips, and your toes are pointing forward. Lift up on the sternum and front of the chest, knowing that posture is important when it comes to relaxing the pelvic floor. If you're hunched over, that's going to engage the pelvic floor, because now the pelvic floor is doing the work of helping your torso stabilize on your pelvis instead of your legs and upper back. Uplift your chest and uplift your eyes, gazing on the horizon or above, keeping your chin parallel with the ground. Allow yourself to stand up straight.

Notice where you feel movement in your body. Maybe you feel your heartbeat pulsing blood through your body, maybe you feel muscles twitching somewhere, maybe you feel your bowels or gas moving around. Simply notice where you feel movement in the body. Pause.

Now notice where you feel stillness. Standing up tall, notice the areas of movement and stillness as you scan your body from the top of your head to the tips of your toes. Pause. Balance your weight on your feet, noticing whether you're leaning more on your toes or on your heels. Try to find that center point so the weight of your body is in the middle of your feet. You can rock back and forth to get a feel for which way you may be leaning. Also notice the difference in pressure between the outside of your feet and the inside of your feet. The soles of your shoes will often tell you where you tend to place the weight of your body. For now, I want you to feel it.

Is there more pressure on the inside of your foot or the outside? You can roll your feet back and forth to get a feel for the difference, and then bring them back to the center. Find that perfect balance on the center of your foot. All the while, remember you're pulling up on your front body and you're pulling down on your back body. Pull up on the thighs, front ribs and the sternum, uplifting the chest and the eyes, while you're imagining pulling down on the back body. Shoulders are rolled back and your "wings" are pointed down toward the sit bones. The sit bones are pointing down, and you're anchoring your heels into the floor.

Now you have this circular movement where you're pulling up on the front body and down the back body. Now, allow your breath to follow that movement. As you breathe in, imagine the energy flowing up, and as you breathe out, imagine the energy going down behind you. Take a few breaths and envision a few cycles of energy flowing up the front and down the back. Remember to check in with balancing the weight of your body on the center of your feet and balancing the weight on both your left and right foot equally.

Doing this in front of a mirror can help you align your pelvis and shoulders and provide neurofeedback to your brain about what good posture can feel like. Breathe in as you pull up, and breathe out as you anchor down. Yoga calls this posture, "tadasana."

Maybe you never before put so much thought into standing, but standing can be a meditation you can do anywhere! Qi Gong and Tai Chi also help you practice mindful posture and movement. Some Qi Gong exercises are similar to the "wiggle" exercise you did earlier in this book as it invites you to loosen your body through bouncing and gentle twists. When it comes to movement, the body follows the brain, and the brain follows the body. Rigid bodies lead to a rigidity in thinking. Practicing gentle bounces and fluid twists help create flexibility and fluidity in the mind. Here is an exercise that is similar to a beginner's exercise in Qi Gong.

EXERCISE

Begin with your feet hip-distanced apart and soften your knees to support your lower back.

- Gently begin bouncing up and down—not intensely—even a subtle bounce can be effective. Do this for about two minutes.

- Now moving into a gentle twist, allow your arms to swing front to back. A twist not only provides bilateral stimulation to the brain, it also increases circulation in the brain and around the spine.

- As you're allowing your arms to swing, allow the front hand to reach up and thump on the K27 acupressure points, or the "collarbone" point in EFT. Allow the hand that's in the back to thump on the side of the lower back, which is the kidney point. Stimulating both points increases circulation and helps get the lymphatic system flowing, especially in the pelvic region. Twist and thump on these points for about one to two minutes. Keep your knees soft.

- Now return to just twisting and swinging your arms gently, slowing down the pace.

- Now stand still and notice where you feel movement, buzzing, and/or stillness in your body.

- Take a deep breath in and enjoy a long, slow exhalation. Great job!

Frequency: The Thread of the Universe

Now that your brain is primed and ready to receive more information, let's talk about frequencies. Frequencies are real. They can be measured by scientific instruments. The physical body creates frequencies. The nervous system operates on electrical signals. Your mind operates on electromagnetic currents. Your heartbeat has a frequency, one that inspires it to beat, and one that it creates with different emotions. Your brain creates electromagnetic waves that can be measured by EEG devices and fMRI scans. Transcranial Magnetic Stimulation (TMS) uses magnets to balance and stimulate these frequencies in the brain. Your energy centers of the chakras, also called the "biofield" by the National Institutes of Health, can be measured.

Some people, like Donna Eden*, are blessed with a gift to be able to see this energy with the naked eye. Acupuncture works to balance the energy flows in the meridian system, which is basically like our own personal fiber optic network. Even though you can't see these frequencies, we know they exist and they offer an important access point for healing.

Electromagnetic energy was originally identified by a Scottish physicist names James Clerk Maxwell. He published his findings in 1861 with his equations describing the behavior of electric and magnetic fields. His work eventually lead to the development of people wearing magnets to help soothe motion sickness and arthritis. You can purchase these types of bracelets at your local pharmacy, did you know that? Basically, know this: **You are made of energy. Therefore, you're going to be affected by other electromagnetic systems around you.**

Agitating Frequencies

Electromagnetic frequency radiation (EMF radiation) is created by your Wi-Fi equipment, computers, and cell phones. There has been an increase in awareness around the development of tumors and associated cancers due to cell phones and wireless Bluetooth headphones.

---

* Visit www.edenmethod.com for more information about Donna.

There are so many EFT radiation frequencies that are always around you that are affecting your system and you don't even realize it.

On the other hand, when you have a history of trauma or history of chronic pain, your system becomes more sensitive and more tuned in to all of these other subtle frequencies. This can be a blessing and a curse. It can be a blessing because you become aware of it and you can really tune it down and turn it down. On the other hand, these intrusive frequencies, including 4G and 5G networks, can increase your sensitivity levels and increase your systemic inflammation. If you experience Lyme disease, autoimmune issues, or dysautonomia, your system is more sensitive to the frequencies around you. Some of my clients experience vagal reactions when they're around too many electronics and when they're around a large power source, such as the powerful electrical box on the telephone pole. Understanding how your biological systems are affected by things like this can help you start to make sense of your "strange" experiences and you can learn to adjust your lifestyle accordingly. Here is a short list of things you can purchase to help support your body when you're surrounded by a lot of these electronic frequencies.

- Copper balls and copper jewelry. Copper is still used in every grounded electrical outlet. Some Reiki practitioners use copper balls and large copper spirals under their treatment tables to help ground the energy of both practitioner and patient.
- DefenderShield is a popular brand of EMF protective equipment.

Healing Frequencies

The frequency of sound and light offer our bodies healing on a level that can't be touched or influenced by a person. Let's start with talking about sound.

The nervous system is an electromagnetic system, and it matches the frequency of the sound that is around you. Sound therapy uses singing bowls and tuning forks to gently guide the nervous system into a harmonized frequency. Binaural music—or bilateral stimulation music—

utilizes a similar concept in that the composers choose specific sounds, tones, and rhythms that feel peaceful to the nervous system.

When you're feeling agitated, you can become aware of the sounds surrounding you, and ask yourself if they could be adding to your nervous systems' agitation. Think about different types of music. Your nervous system responds differently if it's hard rock, heavy metal, pop, or classical. The different instruments create different types of frequencies and tones that can either calm or agitate the nervous system.

Sound, and specifically music, is stored all over the brain. When you play music, your brain lights up everywhere, even in the sensory-motor cortex. Research demonstrates the power of music to inspire Parkinson's patients to be able to dance as well as calm their systems, when before they would have uncontrollable and jerky movements. Connie Tomiano, with the Institute for Music and Neurologic Function at Beth Abraham Health Services in the Bronx, New York, says "For people who have motor problems, music acts as a catalyst. Hearing a beat can be enough to carry a person from thinking to moving." Similarly, stroke victims who have sensory-motor problems can use music to "wake up" the brain and "remember" how to move again. Music and sound act as catalysts and help the brain guide the body in moving in ways that weren't thought possible before. Take a moment to view the trailer of an incredible documentary called, "Alive Inside" (available on YouTube). This documentary reviews the power of sound and music in an emotionally moving way.

Ultrasound, which uses sound frequency, is now being used to treat hernias, scar tissue, connective tissue disease, and chronic muscle spasms. Ask your physical therapist if this is an option in their office.

When navigating chronic pain, involuntary neuromuscular activation, and autonomic nervous system upregulation, one can feel powerless over the brain's reactivity. Maybe your mind is racing when trying to listen to a meditation, or a muscle spasm is too intense to focus on breath work. These experiences can make it feel so difficult to calm your nervous system.

Music and sound therapy can be the remedy. The rhythm, speed, volume, and tones affect the nervous system in different ways. Jeffrey Thompson's research on the music he composed demonstrates this, as well as the recently developed Apollo Neuro device by Dr. David Rabin. Both use the power of sound frequency to choose the frequency of the nervous system and "channel" it to whatever mode you desire.

For example, the Apollo Neuro* is a wearable device that you can program to turn on automatically throughout the day, which is very useful when your goal is to heal your autonomic nervous system and chronic pain. The more frequently you calm your nervous system throughout the day, the more easily it will be to calm your system at the end of the day. The device, which delivers vibrations, offers seven different channels: (1) energy and wake up, (2) social and open, (3) clear and focused, (4) rebuild and recover, (5) meditation and mindfulness, and (6) relax and unwind. Pretty amazing, right? It works brilliantly and almost immediately. It's also subtle. If you are in a public space and don't feel comfortable practicing EFT or if you don't have time to do breathing exercises or a meditation, the Apollo Neuro is very convenient. Personally, I have used the Apollo Neuro to successfully titrate off caffeine and it provided me with more sustainable energy. The Apollo Neuro is also very effective at calming my system and preparing me for a deep sleep, which is especially beneficial during those late-night workdays when I want to go straight to sleep rather than needing to "wind down" with an hour of television.

When you have severe dysautonomia, calming the nervous system too quickly can actually cause an abreaction. Remember, anything unfamiliar to the brain is deemed unsafe until proven otherwise. We see this when someone is pulled from freezing water: You can't put them in warm water because the temperature differentiation causes a shock to the system, so even warm water feels scalding hot. I've worked with clients who have had to experiment with different types of instrumental music to find a slower "step-down" process before their nervous systems were able to handle the calming effects of the Apollo Neuro or

---

* www.apolloneuro.com or www.wearablehugs.com

Jeffrey Thompson's music. When music doesn't seem to quite do it for you, return to the power of your own body's instrument: singing.

In the book *The Healing Power of Sound*, author Mitchell Gaynor, MD, reports that sound has the ability to reduce anxiety, reduce heart and respiratory rates, reduce cardiac complications, lower blood pressure, increase immune cell messengers, decrease stress hormones during medical testing, and boost natural opiates—all extremely useful for healing chronic pain! In his book, he reviews a variety of ways you can use your voice and various vocal sounds to initiate healing in various areas of your body. One of my favorite exercises is to sing all of the vowel sounds and allow the sound to last as long as possibe. This naturally lengthens the exhalation, which, as I've already discussed, aids in calming the vagus nerve and autonomic nervous system. Let's practice.

EXERCISE: SING THE VOWELS

Inhale completely and create the following sounds, one at a time, allowing each sound to last as long as possible. Notice where you feel the different vowel sounds in your body.

- "Ah"
- "Eh"
- "Eeee"
- "Ohhh"
- "Oooo"
- Now, repeat those sounds at a lower or higher pitch and notice where you feel the physical sensation move in your body.

MY HEART'S SONG

I've always enjoyed singing. Ancestrally, I imagine it would be hard not to. While I fantasized about being on stage leading the high school musical, I also became frozen stiff on the stage, despite my 10+ years of ballet performances. I'll always remember my first night as the "narrator" in "Joseph and the Technicolored Dreamcoat" when I completely forgot my lines and the choir director glared at me. When I got off stage my teacher said, "I'm so sorry the mics went out!" It turned out only me and the choir director knew I had forgotten the lines. According to everyone else, the mics stopped working. Ha! Needless to say, the choir director didn't let me forget.

The point of that story was my attempt at celebrating a moment of being human. The real story I want to share is how singing saved me. No, it didn't save me from the emotional pain of humiliation during the high school musical. It did, however, save me from physical pain when I was in labor with a broken pelvis. I had fallen when I was six months' pregnant thanks to my wrist being tied around the leash when my dog decided to chase a rabbit. My physician thought I was overreacting to "normal pubic symphysis pain" during pregnancy. My midwife wouldn't admit anything, but her face, when she examined me, said enough. "Keep up with the squats, and you'll be fine," she said. "Gee, thanks," I thought. It wasn't until three months after my child was born when I was able to go to a colleague for evaluation and she confirmed that my pelvis was cracked, one side was shifted forward, and part of my inner adductor muscle had pulled so hard off the bone that a bone chip was floating and hanging off a part of the ligament right below my pubic symphysis. "Ouch," she said as she moved the ultrasound machine around.

Yeah, I sang a lot that year. Every time I had to use my pelvis—and as you already know, you use your pelvis for everything—I sang. It was the only way I could keep breathing through the pain, and function through the pain. That's the year I *really* learned what it was like to manage pelvic floor dysfunction. I learned that the internal obturator is stubborn—so is the piriformis. I had to work through my anger toward my body for "failing me," and shift to a place of gratitude that it sustained three months of pregnancy on a broken pelvis. I actually had pimples on all of the tapping points on my face because I was tapping so much!

What was most amazing to me was how the gaze of my infant's eyes gave me amnesia for sensation in my body. In that moment, it was pure love, pure spirit, pure peace. That's the power of love. That's the power of the heart's song.

I invite you to discover your heart's song in this moment. What makes your heart sing?

Light Therapy

Photobiomodulation, better known as light therapy, has many uses and powerful effects on the physical body. Light therapy is normalized when it comes to babies with jaundice and getting rid of those pesky wrinkles. However, it's only recently gaining mainstream momentum in the treatment of chronic pain. One company, SoLa, has created a wand that looks like an intravaginal ultrasound device. This wand brings red light and near-infrared light to the internal muscles via the vaginal canal. It's currently only FDA approved for vaginal access, but they are trying to get FDA approval for rectal access so male CPP patients can benefit as well.

The good news is that with most red light and near-infrared lights, the light frequency is powerful enough to permeate up to 2 to 3 inches deep when held 6 inches from the body. Therefore, depending on your size, a red light therapy device shining on your front and your back could arguably cover your entire body inside and out. Red light and near-infrared light have been shown to speed up the regeneration of nerve cells, muscle cells, and connective tissue and even help with organ repairs by decreasing inflammation. Here is a list of current applications of photobiomodulation, according to Hamblin and Huang (2013, CRC Press):

- Hair regrowth
- Tinnitus
- Skin rejuvenation
- Neck pain
- Unsealed fractures
- Arthritis
- Wound healing
- Stroke
- Traumatic brain injury (including concussions)
- Temporomanidubular join disorder (TMJ)
- Dental pain
- Chronic pain
- Mucositis

- Reduction of myocardial infarction
- Lateral epicondylitis
- Carpal tunnel syndrome
- Muscle fatigue
- Achilles tendonitis

From looking at this list, you can ascertain that light therapy can be good for everyone and just about everything. I've even used it to speed up healing for my pets' wounds. One time, when my cat needed a major leg surgery due to getting attacked by a fox, the vet said she required full limitation of movement for three weeks. How do you keep an outside cat in a crate for three weeks?! I used light therapy on her, and she was fully healed within a week and a half. The vet was shocked and bought a red light for their veterinarian rehabilitation office. Light therapy can certainly be helpful for the whole family!

Photobiomodulation works in a variety of ways, but one of the main things it does is increase the energy that the molecules create inside the cells. I spoke briefly in an earlier chapter about our emotions' effects on water molecules. Light frequency basically speeds up the rotor of the molecule's engine to create more "ATP"—the power units essential to innumerable metabolic processes in living cells.

Different light frequencies help with different things. See the graphs below, taken from *Light Therapies: A Complete Guide to the Healing Power of Light* by Anadi Martel. The different colors permeate at different depths and cause different effects for cardiac health and emotional health.

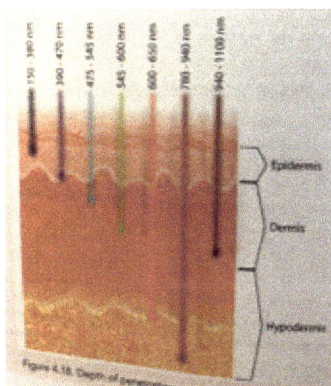

©Sensortech

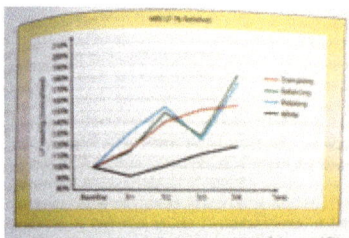
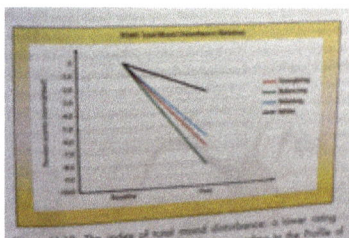

©Sensortech

It's ideal if you can find a lamp that has the whole spectrum, including the blue and yellow (which also gives you green) as well as the red, infrared, and near infrared. Light therapy can help with brain chemistry balancing and mood regulation, including the resolution of depression, anxiety, and insomnia, in as few as six sessions—with *no negative side effects*.

Light therapy has the potential to help with all significant triggers of CPP, including reducing inflammation in the bladder and GI system and reducing the growth of, and nerve damage from, endometriosis and neuropathies. Things like persistent genital arousal disorder (PGAD) and bladder urgency are extremely distressing to live with. If photobiomodulation could help cure these conditions without needing the invasive and painful treatments of nerve injections, how amazing would that be?! We need more funding for research in this area of medicine, but I don't think we're too far behind that possibility. Thank you, SoLa!

Here's how you can help address the pudendal nerve and sometimes the genito-femoral nerve and the illiohypogastric nerve—all major players in chronic pelvic and sexual pain. This light placement can address all of the nerves in the saddle area, the genital region, and even some of the deeper layers of the vagina, due to the depth of the red and near-infrared light permeation. You may be asking, "How do I get light therapy were the sun doesn't shine?" Well, I've positioned my big teddy bear to demonstrate:

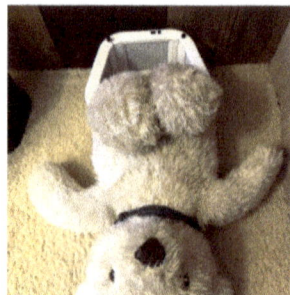

Simply place the light against the wall, remove clothing—the light must shine on bare skin—and place your legs up the wall or rest them on a chair, lie back, and relax! I often listen to a meditation or practice my breathing exercises during my daily 10-minute light therapy routines.

Always remember to wear protective eye goggles! All light therapy lamps come with protective glasses, and if they don't, question the legitimacy of the company and the lamp. You could also do another 10 minutes on your face and you can not only improve your complexion (bonus!), but also balance the brain activity and improve circulation.

Rainbows Heal the Brain

Let's talk a little bit more about the cognitive aspects of light and color. Earlier in this book, I mentioned the healing power of walking in nature because of the colors and the patterns. Well, I'm going to repeat that here. When healing the brain and balancing the nervous system, you need to think about the amount of color in your environment. I remember the first time I started working with someone virtually during COVID whom I had only seen in my office. During the telehealth visits, I noticed there was zero color in their entire house. All of the walls were an off-white color, and the furniture was dark gray. Even the framed images on the wall were in black-and-white. I thought to myself, "Well, this certainly isn't helping their depression."

Most people are familiar with the diagnosis of Seasonal Affective Disorder, which is attributed to the lack of sunlight exposure and a dramatic decrease in environmental colors during the winter months (assuming you live above or below a certain latitude around the globe). Research demonstrates a significant change in cerebral blood flow when someone stares at a colorful image versus a gray-scale image. Therefore, when the goal is brain healing, we want to increase blood flow. Bring on the colorful kaleidoscopes! Actually, research shows that when people are looking through a colorful kaleidoscope, it has the power to put the brain into theta brainwaves, which demonstrates a deep relaxation.

Exposure to fractals, or symmetrical patters in nature, are also healing for the brain. The Japanese call it "forest bathing." There's also research from Australia that demonstrates people heal faster from surgeries when their hospital rooms have a view of nature versus buildings. Next time you find yourself in the hospital, request a room with trees as the backdrop or spend some money on a lot of plants to look at while you're there.

Light, Melatonin, and Circadian Rhythms

Our brains also follow the daylight to create what's called the circadian rhythm. Certainly now that many humans are spending their lives inside, rather than outside, this affects everyone at some level. Your circadian rhythm can become out of balance with chronic pain because of how that affects your cortisol levels.

You can see this more significantly depending on what shift you work. If you tend to work second shift or third shift, that can create disruptions in your circadian rhythm, which then disturbs your sleep cycle. Once you disturb sleep, things really start getting out of balance.

In order to help reset your circadian rhythm, you need to manage the light that is around you during the day. I learned the following routine from an integrative medicine physician: For three weeks, watch the sunrise and the sunset. The light frequencies change as the sun is going up or down on the horizon due to the shifting angle at which the light hits the atmosphere. That's why the sun looks different colors during sunrise and sunset. As the light enters your brain, it aids turning on or off the brain's natural development of melatonin.

If you feel this is true for you, be ready to watch the sunrise or sunset for five minutes before and 10 minutes after so your brain observes the full spectrum change. Someone may ask, "What if it's cloudy out?" Well, the beautiful thing about light frequency is that it goes through the clouds. 😊 If you work during the hours of sunrise or sunset, then an at-home light therapy lamp is ideal for you.

Also, keep in mind the blue light emitted from your screens. Thanks to the widespread awareness of the research in the past few years, many TVs, computers, and phones now come with a built-in blue-light filter. If you don't have one, you can purchase blue light-blocking eyeglasses and filters for your screens. The blue light stops your brain from creating its own melatonin. Melatonin is necessary for a healthy circadian rhythm, and many other healing functions of the body.

A Few Notes on Melatonin

If you've ever utilized melatonin to sleep, know that it only is effective in *helping* the brain during short-term use. After 10 days, the brain will stop creating its own melatonin. Consequently, if used long-term, when you stop using melatonin your brain goes through withdrawal and has difficulty falling asleep and staying asleep. Most people think this is evidence that melatonin was working for them. Unfortunately, it was creating a problem.

Melatonin is very effective for people traveling for work and needing help rebalancing jetlag. It can also be helpful for people who have switching day-night shifts and need help resetting their internal clocks. However, try not to use it for more than 10 days. If you are a long-time user, I recommend working with a trusted healthcare provider to begin titrating off of melatonin. I often recommend using herbal teas like Kava tea or Rhodiola Rosea tea in combination with any of the mindfulness meditations and exercises discussed throughout this book. Again, light therapy can help significantly.

Brain-produced melatonin also helps balance the cortisol and oxytocin and other metabolites and hormones that are important for neural activity and systemic health. In his book, *Becoming Supernatural*, Joe Dispenza lists the following scientific facts about melatonin.

- Stops the excess secretion of cortisol in response to stress
- Improves carbohydrate metabolism
- Lowers triglyceride levels
- Inhibits atherosclerosis (hardening of the arteries)

- Heightens the immune response (cellular and metabolic)
- Decreases the development of certain tumors
- Increases lifespan in laboratory rats by 25 percent
- Activates a neuroprotective role in the brain
- Increases REM sleep (dream sleep)
- Stimulates free radical scavenging (anti-aging, antioxidant)
- Promotes DNA repair and replication

Recent research demonstrates that even a faint light in your bedroom will actually keep your brain from getting into that deeper level of sleep. So if you're a fan of nightlights (as are many trauma survivors), **you can keep the nightlight but wear an eye mask.**

A Few More Fun Facts to Think About

As someone who experiences chronic inflammation, chronic pain, and a history of trauma, your system is more sensitive to subtle changes in the atmosphere, including solar flares, storm systems, and shifts in the magnetic poles. If solar flares can take out satellites (yes, that happens), think of what it could do to your biofield and nervous system. Check out the correlation of solar flares and historical events in the graph below.

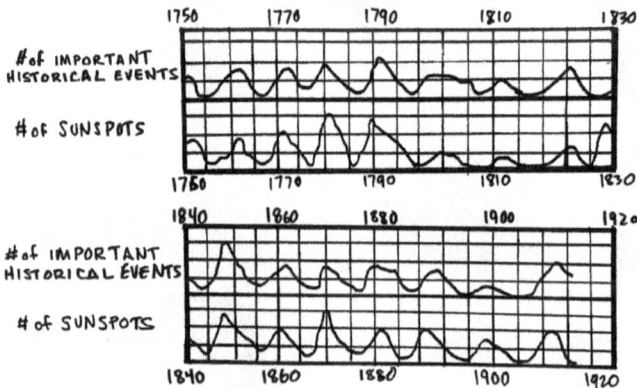

CORRELATION BETWEEN SOLAR ACTIVITY AND HUMAN EVENTS

This is an illustration of a graph that was created from data provided in the translation of Tchijevsky's paper "Physical Factors of the Historical Process" (Tchijevsky, 1971). In the graph, the number of important historical events is plotted in blue on top, the number of sunspots below in red. Alexander Tchijevsky constructed an "Index of Mass Human Excitability" (published in Russian in 1926). The histories of 72 countries were compiled and plotted against the sunspot activity from 1750 to 1922. Tchijevsky found that 80 percent of the most significant human events occurred during the five years of maximum solar activity. He also found that 80 percent of the most significant human events occurred during the five years or so of maximum sunspot activity. A solar maximum can increase human warfare activity, as well as human creativity.

Looking at this, I think anyone can agree that solar flares affect the agitation of our nervous systems. We see similar patterns in relation to the moon cycles. If you have ever worked on a crisis line, in a hospital, or as a first responder, you know to expect a surge in activity around the full moon. I suppose if a full moon can pull an entire ocean into high tide, it would affect the water molecules in our bodies, right? There's even reports on the National Business Aviation Association website for when airports had to repaint the numeric designators at each end of the runway because of the movement of the magnetic poles. We are made of electromagnetic energy; any movement in the magnetic poles of our planet is going to affect us.

I don't claim to have it all figured out. I'm simply sharing some of these interesting facts to give you something to think about the next time you're in a pain flare. There's a lot we can't control when it comes to things that agitate our nervous system, which is exactly why it's important to practice the techniques I've provided you in this book. I want you to feel prepared to soothe your system no matter what revs it up.

Chapter 11

Mind-Body: Connection or Disconnection?

In the summer of 2021, I had the privilege of hearing Dr. Bruce Greyson speak at Chautauqua Institution.* He spoke about his research on near death experiences (NDEs) and how he accidentally fell into this line of focus when his patient reported something astonishing during his early years as a physician in the emergency room. Dr. Greyson started off by highlighting that he grew up a "materialist" and didn't believe in anything but the physical form. His research, however, has led him to challenge his belief system over and over again.

His presentation matched what I've heard from clients over the years who experienced NDEs, and I found his book, *After,* even more validating and fascinating. He shares story after story from interviews all over the world. After 50 years of international research, he states that all NDEs have the following three variables in common: (1) independence from cultural and spiritual expectations, (2) memories are stable over decades, and (3) experiences are called "realer than real." What I love most about what he shares is the evidence demonstrating that **the mind functions independently of the brain.** So, no matter how many traumatic brain injuries you've experienced, you can practice utilizing the power of the mind to overcome many adversities.

Dr. Greyson provides pages of examples of how people have memories of what was going on in the operating room during surgery, even though they were unconscious. I, myself, have heard numerous stories—also

---

*C hautauqua Institution is a summer destination for adults who love to learn, feel intellectually challenged, and have a safe place for their children to play unattended. Check it out at www.chq.org

unchanged over years of seeing the same client. Clients have told me their recollections of events that occurred when they were either unconscious, under sedation, or even temporarily flat-lined. The majority of stories that were told to me were confirmed by other members of their family or their physician.

So, what does this tell us? I think there's a strong case that something in us is always paying attention. I don't claim to know what it is, but I assume **it's all involved: mind, body, heart, and spirit**. Therefore, **even if you don't have a conscious memory of something that happened, your body is remembering and can therefore react to these memories being triggered.**

There is a bridge between the physical and the spiritual realm. Based on Dr. Greyson's research, and the 600 pages of research in *The Irreducible Mind*, by Edward and Emily Williams Kelly, this bridge can be accessed through the mind. This brings me to one of my favorite quotes from Rumi: "I am not this hair. I am not this skin. I am the soul that lives within."

The Difference Between the Mind and the Brain in the Words of a 7-Year-Old

"My mind is telling me to save my money, but my brain is telling me to do the opposite. My brain is telling me to use my allowance money to buy LEGO set. My mind is telling me that I don't need the LEGO set and I should save my money and wait until I *really* want something. My brain is telling me that I *really want and need* the LEGO set *today*." Yes, this is what the internal world sounds like to a child who is raised by a specialist in the mind-body connection! Impressive! (I'm his mother, I can say that. ☺)

This dialogue demonstrates the impulses and perception of the brain based on dopamine-boosting experiences of purchasing a new toy. My son's recognition of the difference between the mind and the brain is what the practice of mindfulness provides. With training, the mind can develop the position of the "observer." As the observer, you can view the brain's visual and auditory displays from a distance and realize that you are not those things. You are the observer. The mind is the observer, and you can change the channel at any time. When your brain feels like an annoying commercial, you can turn it off. Yes, my child. Yes, you can.

A Final Note

Mindfulness invites us to become the observer and guide of our entire system. Mindfulness invites us to realize that our experience does not have to be dictated by thoughts, emotions, physical experience, or generational trauma. All of these can create a tipping point for when part of us reacts and changes directions, but if we practice harnessing the mind, harnessing our ability to observe, recalibrate, and refocus on what we want, then we can strongly control where we're going and who we are becoming. Even if we can't control the weather, we can still control the sails and the rudder. It's worth it, don't you agree?

All of the exercises in this book are aimed at calming the brain's habit of looking at the past and saying, "I don't see any evidence of why I'm going to get better." I hope you use these exercises to neutralize your body's trauma- and fear-based reactions and reprogram your brain. Heal the hardware, and update the software. I believe in you.

Chapter 12

When All Else Fails— A Few "Miracle" Stories

Here's the thing. I know these exercises work. I've seen it, I've experienced it, and I've read the research (like, a LOT of it). Therefore, when I'm working with someone and their symptoms do not improve with these interventions and practices, we're missing something. Sometimes, it's a medical condition that has not been identified. Sometimes it's generational trauma. Sometimes it's our environment. You must have patience, persistence, and compassion. I'd like to share a few success stories about clients I've worked with.

Case 1

One time I was working with someone who was experiencing pain and inflammation all over. She knew that taking an antibiotic significantly decreased her pain and improved her function, but she was unable to access and safely use antibiotics constantly. She had seen more than 20 doctors, with no answers. Then, one day, she set off a security alarm at the airport. She realized the doctors had completed CTs and MRIs, but never an X-ray. When she was able to find a doctor to order one, she "lit up like a Christmas tree." Her entire torso, and even upper thighs, were decorated with titanium and nickel clips from her gallbladder surgery performed more than 20 years earlier. She was allergic to nickel, which she knew, but her surgeon never told her what the clips were made of. Remarkably, she was able to locate a surgeon who agreed to remove as many of the clips as he could find. During this surgery, he confirmed her intuition: she had major layers of infection throughout her abdomen. She isn't pain-free yet. However, her persistence led to the answers and validation she desired, and provided her with a more effective map on how to heal. She now utilizes ionic foot baths to remove the metals floating throughout her body, and many of the interventions discussed in this book to support her ongoing healing.

Case 2

One time I was working with someone who, in addition to CPP, experienced intense panic attacks. However, she didn't present as an anxious person. She would talk about how it "came out of nowhere." We focused treatment on her myriad of unresolved traumatic incidents throughout her upbringing, utilizing all of the techniques in this book. Her trauma-based symptoms ended, but the random panic attacks persisted. After several doctors and many letters from me on her behalf, we were able to get her a Holter monitor for two weeks. It turns out, she had an undiagnosed cardiac condition, which was resolved by a very simple outpatient procedure. She never had another panic attack, and her pelvic floor dysfunction and CPP resolved within two months.

Case 3

One of my favorite things to do in my career is to help women with fertility complications. One woman I worked with had a history of endometriosis, three failed attempts of in vitro fertilization, and was told she would never get pregnant. When she walked the 4-D Wheel, an important connection came to light: she was afraid to become pregnant. Her mother had experienced fertility issues and required the use of a surrogate in order to have her. My client anticipated feeling immense guilt and shame if she was able to become pregnant when her mother was not able to. She went on to describe a codependent, enmeshed relationship with her mother, which means there was a history of feeling responsible for her mother's emotional well-being. Using some of the techniques in this book, we cleared the feelings of responsibility and guilt and shame around her own desire of wanting to experience a healthy and successful pregnancy. She gave birth a year later and went on to have a few more children.

Case 4

One story that relates to the power of brain mapping and secondary trauma occurred when I worked with someone who had pain in the left side of her lower abdomen and had years of painful cysts and fibroids in that part of her body. She also struggled with constipation and "back up" of bowels in that part of her descending colon. Note that according to Chinese medicine, the left side of your body symbolizes the feminine relationships in your life, and the right side of your body symbolizes the masculine relationships in your life. Knowing this, I asked her if she had any relationship issues with her mother. She started to cry. Her childhood was strewn with secondary trauma as she observed her mother going through *left-sided ovarian cancer* in the same location that my client had her pain. During adolescence, she observed her mother going through years of chemo, lying and crying on the couch, in high expressions of pain, and eventually, dying. My client grew up terrified of her reproductive organs and anticipated getting cancer in the same area of her body. After completing trauma work on these experiences and fear, her pain disappeared, and her body stopped creating cysts.

Case 5

One time I was working with someone who had complex post-traumatic stress disorder and a history of a wide variety of psychiatric diagnoses and inpatient hospital stays for mental health. She experienced CPP, nightmares, migraines, and "brain fog," which I later diagnosed as dissociation. After six months of biweekly treatment, her partner joined a session and provided his perspective on her panic attacks. His description detailed rapid eye movements, twitches, and incoherent speech. She had never shared this with me before because she had apparently been experiencing amnesia during these episodes, and they had never talked about it. With those added details, (and again, many letters and pleading with physicians) I was able to find a neurologist to provide a CT scan and EEG. Low and behold, she was not only suffering from a seizure disorder, but her scans showed brain damage from a lifetime of seizures that were undiagnosed and untreated. After four months on medication and continuing her pelvic floor physical therapy (and other exercises in this book), her trauma, anxiety, and CPP symptoms subsided.

Case 6

One time I was working with someone who, in addition to CPP, experienced chronic migraines on one side of her head in a very specific place on her forehead. When the migraine would start, her CPP would flare. Knowing the connection between the vagus nerve and the pelvic floor, I didn't think much of it at first, assuming only a physiological connection. After retraining her brain and nervous system, the symptoms didn't subside. I took a leap of faith one day and asked her to have a conversation with her mother about the specific location and if she (the mother) had experienced any head trauma. The story she told gave us both goosebumps. Her mother shared the story of *her* mother, my client's grandmother, who at age 16 had been kidnapped, raped, and hit on the head. She was found later by neighbors and had talked about it briefly in the last months of her life. We practiced tapping on that experience and her reaction to hearing that story. We then created a guided visualization in which she imagined sending healing to her grandmother. Then, guess what? She never had another migraine.

My point is that you must trust your intuition. Fear and intuition physically feel like they're in the same place—right in the gut—in the center of our solar plexus. That's why it's so important to neutralize fear, so we can **tune into our intuition and dialogue with our bodies** so we can discover what else is going on. I am an absolute "believer" that the body is capable of returning to its natural state of balance, homeostasis, and well-being. I believe because I've seen it. I believe because I understand how the system works. I believe because I've experienced it. *Connect with yourself. Dialogue with your body. Soothe your mind, body, heart, and spirit. You have all the resources you need.*

◀■▶ EXERCISE

On a scale from 1–10 (1 being low, 10 being high), what is your current level of belief and hope about your ability to heal? Write that here:

Did it improve since the starting this book? Circle YES or NO

Now, get out the large 4-D Wheel and place it on the floor. Retrieve the objects you chose at the beginning of this book. Walk the 4-D Wheel with each object. Be curious, explore, and discover the transformations you have experienced by reading this book and going through these exercises.

Take notes, keep walking the Wheel, and never give up.

Breathe. Believe. Be.

Thank you for taking this journey with me.

The resources in the following appendices include those mentioned in the main chapters as well as extra "bonus" material. Please enjoy all of the resources available to you!

Appendix A

Take the Quiz

1. How can pain education help you?
   a. It turns a big scary lion into a baby lion (metaphorically speaking)
   b. It decreases the frequency, duration, and intensity of pain flares
   c. It teaches us how and why we need to retrain the brain to heal painful habits
   d. All of the above

2. What kinds of note-taking are effective?
   a. Doodling
   b. Writing everything down
   c. Drawing images and concepts of things that stand out to you
   d. Any note-taking is better than none
   e. All of the above

3. Brain mapping explains:
   a. Generational trauma
   b. Why our brains react the way they do
   c. Why we experience pain in such individualized ways
   d. All of the above

4. Your brain reacts to:
   a. Real events
   b. Imagined events
   c. Past memories and traumas
   d. Someone telling you a story about their experience
   e. All of the above

5. What happens when your brain's reserve is maxed out?
    a. The nerves become more sensitive
    b. The nervous system stays in "fight/flight/freeze" mode
    c. Physical healing slows down
    d. A smaller stimulus creates a bigger response
    e. All of the above

6. You can help your brain neutralize past traumas and associated thoughts and beliefs.
    a. True
    b. False

7. What are some exercises that help decrease and neutralize negative thoughts?
    a. Emotional Freedom Techniques (EFT)
    b. REBT chart
    c. Byron Katie's 4 questions
    d. Brainspotting
    e. All of the above

8. Thoughts and beliefs create a frequency that affect how your autonomic nervous system functions.
    a. True
    b. False

9. The founder of physical therapy said "our issues are in our tissues." Therefore, healing emotional wounds and trauma is necessary to heal chronic pain.
    a. True
    b. False

10. Our emotions emit a frequency that changes the molecular structure and function of our bodies.
    a. True
    b. False

11. The STOP procedure means:
    a. Stop what you're doing and take a nap
    b. Stop complaining and deal with it
    c. Stop, take a breath, observe, proceed
    d. Stop in the name of love

12. Brain research demonstrates that ___ minutes a day of mindfulness heals the brain's hardware within 21 days.
    a. 5
    b. 10
    c. 15
    d. 20

13. Practicing mindfulness and bilateral stimulation daily can heal the hardware of the brain within 21 days:
    a. True
    b. False

14. Practicing the following counts as mindfulness practice:
    a. "I spy" with all five senses
    b. Playing an instrument
    c. Having intentional attention during your physical therapy exercises and stretches
    d. Slowly enjoying one bite of food
    e. All of the above

15. Which of the following is meditative mindfulness, versus active mindfulness?
    a. Progressive muscle relaxation
    b. Breathing exercises
    c. Guided visualization
    d. "I spy" with all five senses

16. Compassion and empathy are two separate neural circuits in the brain.
    a. True
    b. False

17. Which of the following increases oxytocin (the bliss/healing hormone)?
    a. Physical touch
    b. Eye contact
    c. Social support
    d. Orgasm
    e. All of the above

18. Which of the following exercises heals the hardware of your brain?
    a. Bilateral stimulation
    b. Mindfulness-based stress reduction
    c. Healing the GI system
    d. Breathing exercises
    e. All of the above

19. Pain is a signal generated by the brain, not the body.
    a. True
    b. False

20. Pain means there is tissue damage somewhere.
    a. True
    b. False

21. The brain only responds to things that are true in the moment. It never responds to things from the past or the future.
    a. True
    b. False

22. GI health influences brain health.
    a. True
    b. False

23. Our nervous system matches the frequency of sound in the environment.
    a. True
    b. False

24. Our emotions emit a frequency that changes the molecular structure and function of our bodies.
    a. True
    b. False

25. Tapping (EFT) not only calms the nervous system, it also helps your brain neutralize and file away fear-based thoughts and images.
    a. True
    b. False

26. The breath is the only part of the autonomic nervous system that you can gain conscious control over.
    a. True
    b. False

27. You can heal the "garden of your mind" with compassionate curiosity, imagining the life you want, and relaxation.
    a. True
    b. False

28. The most important part of creating positive affirmations is:
    a. You must FEEL it for it to be effective
    b. It sounds good to others
    c. Someone else wrote it
    d. It's the opposite of what you believe currently

29. What's the best way to develop a self-care routine?
    a. Routine: same time daily, ideally 2x/day
    b. Gradual increase: start with 5 minutes and increase by 5 minutes weekly
    c. Reward: reward yourself after your practice and after you achieve a personal goal
    d. Reminder: set reminders for yourself
    e. Remember: there's no failure, only feedback
    f. All of the above

30. What activity helps (re)create trust and intimacy in a relationship?
    a. Eye gazing
    b. Sensate-focused touch
    c. Breath work
    d. Waiting for spontaneous desire
    e. A, B, and C

ANSWER KEY: 1D, 2E, 3D, 4E, 5E, 6A, 7E, 8A, 9A, 10A, 11C, 12D, 13A, 14E, 15C, 16A, 17E, 18E, 19A, 20B, 21B, 22A, 23A, 24A, 25A, 26A, 27A, 28A, 29F, 30E

Appendix B

Meditation Scripts

Breathing Exercises

The following breathing exercises gently guide the autonomic nervous system (ANS) back into the parasympathetic, or resting, state. By practicing these techniques on a daily basis, you not only increase the relaxation response in your body, but you also create new habitual patterns of breathing on a regular basis. When your nervous system is habituated to be in the relaxation response, you decrease symptoms of fear, anxiety, depression, and pain. The relaxation response also increases your body's natural healing response.

Begin all breathing exercises by finding a comfortable position, sitting or lying down, where your chest can rest comfortably in an open posture.

Bumblebee Breath

1. Inhale completely through your nose.
2. Exhale through the nose while making a "mmmmmmmm" sound like a bumblebee; allow the exhalation to last as long as possible.
3. Repeat five times.
4. Sound healing option: You can choose a different vowel sound each time (ah, ee, eye, oh, oo).

3-part Inhale

Allow the inhalation to take three parts, breathing into the lower ribs (Step 1), middle ribs (Step 2), and upper ribs (Step 3).

1. Breathe in for 1 count, pause.
2. Breathe in for 1 count, pause.

3. Breathe in for 1 count, pause.
4. Exhale completely.
5. Repeat.

3-part Exhale

Allow the exhalation to take three parts.

1. Inhale completely.
2. Exhale for 1 count, pause.
3. Exhale for 1 count, pause.
4. Exhale for 1 count, pause.
5. Repeat.

Breath Hold

1. Take a deep breath and hold it for 5 seconds.
2. Exhale half of the breath and hold for 5 seconds.
3. Exhale completely and hold for 5 seconds.
4. Inhale halfway and hold for 5 seconds.
5. Breathe normally for about 5 seconds.

Note: Half-breaths in or out are approximate; there is no precise halfway point.

1–5 Count

For use during an anxiety or panic attack.

1. Inhale for 1 count.
2. Exhale for 1 count.
3. Repeat steps 1–2, increasing the count by one each time, until you get to five counts in and five counts out.
4. If having difficulty reaching five counts easily, repeat each count twice before increasing.

Diaphragmatic Breathing

1. Focus your attention on the center of your belly, behind your navel.
2. Breathe in and out, deeply and slowly, a few times. Pull the air all

the way down into your abdomen. Allow the belly to rise and fall naturally. Don't try to make anything happen. Simply allow the breathe to move in and out of your body. Use your imagination to guide the breath deep into the abdomen.

3. Keep breathing, deeply and slowly. Follow your breath as it flows in through your nose, down your throat, into and through your lungs, and into your belly. Keep following it as it flows back out again. (You won't actually pull air into your belly, of course, but it will feel that way.)
4. Continue breathing this way for four to five minutes.
5. Stop and notice what you experience in your body.

Mindful Eating Script

I would like you to focus on a raisin and just imagine that you have never seen anything like it before. Imagine you have just dropped in from Mars at this moment and you have never seen anything like this food before in your life.

With at least a 10-second pause between phrases, and at a slow but deliberate pace, do the following:

Take the raisin and hold it in the palm of your hand, or between your fingers and thumb. **(Pause)**

Pay attention and really see it. **(Pause)**

Look at it carefully, as if you had never seen such a thing before. **(Pause)**

Turn it over between your fingers. **(Pause)**

Explore its texture between your fingers. **(Pause)**

Examine the highlights where the light shines... the darker hollows in any folds. (**Pause**)

Let your eyes explore every part of it, as if you had never seen such a thing before. **(Pause)**

If, while you are doing this, any thoughts come to mind about "what a strange thing we are doing" or "what is the point of this" or "I don't like this," then just note those thoughts and bring your awareness back to the food. **(Pause)**

Now smell the raisin, take it and hold it beneath your nose, and with each breath in, carefully notice the smell of it. **(Pause)**

Now take another look at it. **(Pause)**

Now slowly take the raisin to your mouth, maybe noticing how your hand and arm know exactly where to put it, perhaps noticing your mouth watering as the food comes up. **(Pause)**

Then gently place the raisin in your mouth, noticing how it is "received," without biting it, just exploring the sensations of having it in your mouth. **(Pause)**

And when you are ready, very consciously take a bite into it and notice the tastes that it releases. **(Pause)**

Slowly chewing it,... Noticing the saliva in your mouth,... The change in consistency of the food. **(Pause)**

Then, when you feel ready to swallow, see if you can first detect the intention to swallow as it comes up, so that even this is experienced consciously before you actually swallow it. **(Pause)**

Finally, see if you can follow the sensations of swallowing it, sensing it moving down to your stomach, and also realizing that your body is now exactly one raisin heavier.

Contemplative Meditation Exercise

You can find a demonstration of this exercise at my website: www.dralexmilspaw.com/books/hellodownthere

Ideas for Objects of Contemplation

- External peaceful focus (visual) – light or candle flame
- External peaceful focus (auditory) – music, ventilation

- External peaceful focus (kinesthetic) – temperature of the air, the feeling of the air moving, your clothes against your skin
- Internal peaceful focus (visual) – a favorite memory
- Internal peaceful focus (auditory) – a favorite song, a memory of a loving voice, peaceful hissing in the ears
- Internal peaceful focus (kinesthetic) – your breath, the feeling of peaceful relaxation in your body
- Internal peaceful focus (digital past) – a verbal description to yourself of a pleasant experience you have had (example, thinking about a great vacation)
- Internal peaceful focus (digital present) – a favorite thought, concept, mental construct (example, a mathematical proof)
- Internal peaceful focus (digital future) – the mental anticipation of a future event described in words (example, thinking about a future vacation)

Forest Bathing: Benefits to Spending Time in Nature

The Japanese call it "forest bathing." Research demonstrates that nature provides sounds and visual symmetrical patterns that guide our brains and bodies back to their natural state of well-being. The following research findings are adapted from *The Nature Fix* by Florence Williams.

- After five minutes in a forest surrounded by trees, the heart rate slows, facial muscles relax, and the prefrontal cortex quiets
- Water and birdsong improve mood and alertness
- Spending 15 minutes in nature can reduce levels of the stress hormone cortisol
- Spending time in natural landscapes increases alpha waves in the brain, which are associated with calm and alertness
- Spending an hour-and-a-half in nature reduces rumination and helps us to be less preoccupied with problems
- Spending two hours per week in nature can make us happier and boost overall health and well-being

Glove Anesthesia and Pain Relief*

Perhaps one of the best-known applications of hypnosis is its ability to control pain, whether during chemical anesthetic-free dentistry and major surgery or childbirth, as well as to bring relief from chronic major pain or occasional minor aches and pains, to promote fast healing of wounds, to control bleeding, and for emergency first aid. It is based on the premise that what one thinks and feels, both consciously and sub-consciously, influences what actually happens in the body. Cognitive mental control over blood flow and temperature of the body has been scientifically proven. Directing our thoughts and imagination gives us amazing control over most involuntary body functions, so that we can make parts of the body warm or cool, relaxed or tense, release blockages, salivate, etc. at will. In fact, when a person inadvertently bumps the elbow or knee and immediately gives the body the command "no hurt, no hurt," pain and bruising are bypassed. So too, therapeutic hypnosis can achieve miracles through "mind over matter," relaxation, visualizations, suggestion, and physiological positive response.

Pain is basically the reaction or response to feelings or sensations that are perceived to be hurting in overwhelming, unbearable, and intolerable ways. The human body handles these perceptions in its inner pharmacy by making its own biochemical, morphine-like endorphins to reduce and block pain, preventing the pain-triggering signals from getting to the brain. Hypnosis, with its emphasis on relaxation, sets up a defense against pain, since the more tense a person is, the more aware they are of the pain, and the more they hurt. However, the more relaxed they are and the more they keep their attention focused elsewhere, the more they can control their perceptions of pain, and the less the pain seems to bother them.

Glove anesthesia is important as the traditional method for quick pain relief and reduction of discomfort, because the numbness created in the hand can be so readily transferred from hand to hand and then transferred to any part of the body needed to numb and control the pain sensations or to help someone else. Once you become adept at this skill,

---

*Adapted by Charlie Curtis © 2012 NLP Training Class; reprinted with permission.

you can immediately just command or direct the hand to feel the extreme cold and numb, and the sensation comes and can be used as desired or needed. However, it works best when you take a deep breath and relax a moment first.

Glove Anesthesia to Develop Our Healing Hands

1. Relax where you are by taking several slow, deep breaths. Feet flat on the floor. Close your eyes. Start out with your hands in your lap.
2. Deepen the relaxation, using any method you wish.
3. Imagine there is a buck of ice water by the side of your chair.
4. Place your hand (either one is okay) in the buck of ice water by letting your arm hang down over the side of the chair.
5. Feel the icy cold water and the ice cubes or cracked ice in the bucket.
6. Remember some other time when you had your hands in ice-cold water. Recall just how cold and numb your fingers and hands felt in the ice water.
7. Now make your hand feel just as numb as it did then.
8. Keep your hand in the ice water until it gets more numb, maybe two to three minutes.
9. Take your hand out of the bucket and test it for numbness by pinching it.
10. With your numb hand, touch the sore or painful area (or rub it with your numb hand or even move that hand in a circular motion one to two inches above the painful area).
11. Instruct the subconscious mind to move the numbness from your numb hand into the tender or sore area and to relieve the pain.
12. Rub your hand and tell it to resume a normal feeling. End the session, feeling much better than before, with pain relief (or other result) achieved.

Options: This may also be used to remove certain creative mental blocks by placing the numb hand on the head or forehead area, while giving the subconscious mind the appropriate directions, like "find the best solution," or "guide me to the right ideas," or "give me the energy and motivation needed to accomplish this project well."

Appendix C

Worksheets

The 4-D Wheel of Sexual Experience
by Gina Ogden, Ph.D.

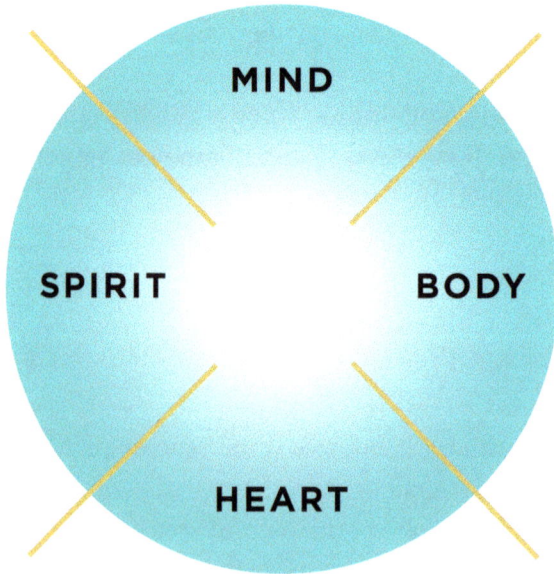

Used with permission from *Exploring Desire and Intimacy: A Workbook for Creative Clinicians* by Gina Ogden. Routledge © 2017.

4D Wheel Worksheet

Utilizing the 4D Wheel to Deepend and Clarify Your Experience

MENTAL: "I think..."

_____
_____
_____
_____
_____
_____
_____
_____
_____
_____
_____

PHYSICAL: "I sense..."

_____
_____
_____
_____
_____
_____
_____
_____
_____
_____
_____

EMOTIONAL: "I feel…"

_____
_____
_____
_____
_____
_____
_____
_____
_____
_____
_____
_____

SPIRITUAL: "I connect…"

_____
_____
_____
_____
_____
_____
_____
_____
_____
_____
_____

"The Shadow Quadrants"

Setting intentions for what you want to change or release from your experience

MENTAL: List at least 3 thoughts, beliefs, or knowledge you want to change or release as part of your therapeutic journey.

_____
_____
_____
_____

PHYSICAL: List at least 3 physical sensations you want to change or release as part of your therapeutic journey.

_____
_____
_____
_____

EMOTIONAL: List at least 3 emotions you want to change or release as part of your therapeutic journey.

_____
_____
_____
_____

SPIRITUAL: List at least 3 connections you want to change or release as part of your therapeutic journey.

_____
_____
_____
_____

"The Light Quadrants"

Setting intentions for what you want to strengthen or invite into your experience

MENTAL: List at least 3 thoughts, beliefs, or knowledge you want to strengthen or invite into your experience.

_____
_____
_____
_____

PHYSICAL: List at least 3 physical sensations you want to strengthen or invite into your experience.

_____
_____
_____
_____

EMOTIONAL: List at least 3 emotions you want to strengthen or invite into your experience.

_____
_____
_____
_____

SPIRITUAL: List at least 3 connections you want to strengthen or invite into your experience.

_____
_____
_____
_____

Activity Record Form

Record on the Activity Record Form each time you practice. Also, make a note of anything that comes up so you can learn which exercises work best for you.

Day/Date	Exercise(s)	Comments
Date/time:		
Date/time:		
Date/time:		
Date/time:		
Date/time:		
Date/time:		
Date/time:		
Date/time:		

Form for Guided Visualization to Your Perfect Place*

1. Select a relaxing, peaceful place, ideally outdoors.

2. Write a short word picture of the scene of your perfect place (real or imagined) to help you remember the details of the scene more strongly.
   a. Where were you?
   b. When did this take place?
   c. What was the weather?
   d. Who was with you, or were you alone?
   e. What was happening around you?
   f. What were you doing?

3. Pick out some sensory details of the memory that were particularly relaxing to you.
   a. Sights
   b. Scents
   c. Sounds
   d. Sensations
   e. Tastes
   f. Emotional feelings

4. Write down any specific sights, sounds, or other sensations that you found particularly peaceful and relaxing.

5. Sit or lie down, and list to the recording.

6. Record your results. 🌳 Visit my website to enjoy the "Guided visualization to your perfect place."

Relationship Communication Charts

List your feelings, behaviors, and values in each column.

YES	MAYBE	NO
(I definitely want and need this.)	**(I could take it or leave it, not a big deal.)**	**(I definitely do NOT want this. This feels like a deal breaker.)**
EXAMPLES: Financial security, trust, honesty, integrity, respect…	Crazy sports fan, eats ice cream late at night…	Racist, sexist, alcoholic, disrespectful…

*Adapted with permission from Charlie Curtis © 2012 NLP Training Class.

Recognizing the power struggle in the relationship

I don't like it when you… (insert partner's behavior)	It makes me feel…(insert emotion)	And I react by… (insert your behavior)	To hide my fear of…
			Not being a good enough partner for you
EXAMPLE: Tell me I'm not doing something right	Ashamed, hurt, sad	Shutting down, leaving the room, giving you the silent treatment	

Recognizing what feels effective and good in the relationship

I like it when you...(insert partner's behavior)	It makes me feel... (insert emotion)	And I respond by... (insert your behavior)	In hopes that you will feel... (insert emotion)
	Nurtured and taken care of	Giving you a hug	Loved and cared for
EXAMPLE: Bring me coffee in the morning			

Relationship and/or Household Meeting Topic Requests

Here is what you can create in a shared notebook or Google doc—giving your partner a heads-up about an issue you want to discuss, and sharing the responsibility to come up with solutions. This increases your readiness to have a conversation, and you can start with solutions rather than criticizing the problem.

Concerns/issues/problems/ things we need to discuss	Possible solutions (list at least 2 for each concern)
EXAMPLE: "Your ADHD makes us late and it stresses out every event we attend."	We can work together on preparation. We can ask for help. We can plan to leave earlier than necessary so we don't feel rushed.

Appendix D
Chakras Related to Pelvic and Sexual Pain

Root Chakra

- Represents foundation
- Function is grounding and elimination
- Fundamental survival needs – food and shelter
- Creates safety and security
- Controls fight or flight
- Connects with spiritual energies of ancestors, their challenges, and their triumphs
- Carries ancestral memories, basically challenges or blockages
- Location: Perineal area and just over the edge of the torso front and back
- Physiological connection: adrenals, feet, legs, bones, large intestine, perineal floor
- Psychological balance: basic survival, safety, groundedness, mother, tribe, feminine divine, passion, determination, righteous anger, courage, strength
- Psychological imbalance: scattered energy, eating disorders, anxiety, fear, greed, excessive negativity, insecurity, frustration, resentment, lack of connection to core self, stubbornness

Sacral Chakra

- Represents procreation
- Function is empowerment
- Seat of creative force and emotions
- Houses the hara

- Location of bliss experience
- Mediates the ability to move forward on path of growth
- Location: centered 2 inches (3-4 finger-widths) below the navel
- Physiological connection: womb, genitals, kidney, bladder, low back, gonads
- Psychological balance: creativity, generativity, self-concept, pleasure, sensuality, healthy appetite, joy, vibrancy, tenderness, nurturing, curiosity, independence, healthy boundaries, elation
- Psychological imbalance: jealousy, guilt, emotional isolation, chronic low back problems, arthritis, hip issues, hedonism, rigidity, manipulation, poor social skills, obsession, need for attention, mood swings

Solar Plexus Chakra

- Represents sustenance, willpower, personal responsibility, clarity, and independence
- Function is survival
- Seat of confidence and in control of life choices
- Storage for sensitivity, ambition, and ability to achieve
- "I" shines from here where one feels strength, will, and personal power
- Core
- Location: midway between the navel and the bottom of the sternum
- Physiological connection: pancreas, adrenals, stomach, small intestine, large intestine, liver, gall bladder
- Psychological balance: personal power, control, self-control, self-discipline
- Psychological imbalance: low self-esteem, lack of clear direction, manipulativeness, control issues, lack of ambition, anger, frustration, powerlessness, shame

Muscle Testing Exercises

The subconscious responds to muscle testing, which is discussed in the research of kinesthetics. You can use muscle testing to determine which chakras (and beliefs or emotions) need to be treated for that particular issue and which do not. When muscle testing on yourself, ask yourself a "yes" or "no" question. If the body responds in a strong and balanced way, then the answer is "yes." When the body responds in a weak and unbalanced way, then the answer is "no." In the illustration below, you see a few different ways you can muscle test. In the example using your fingers, try to keep your fingers together strongly while pulling your hands away from each other. If your fingers stay strong and don't let the loop break, then the answer is "yes." If your fingers are "weak" and break apart, then the answer is "no." With the balancing one, ask someone to gently push you forward or backward with your legs hip distance apart. If you're able to maintain your balance, then your body is answering "yes." If you're unable to maintain your balance and need to catch yourself from falling, then the answer is "no."

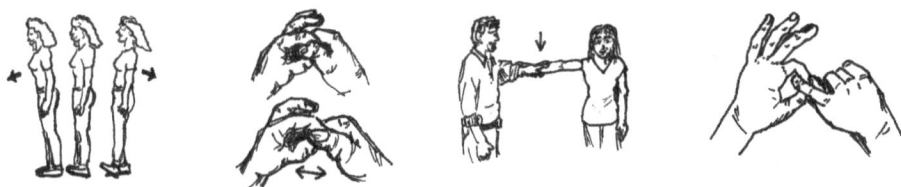

Appendix E

Dr. Milspaw's Recommended Resources*

Recommended Listening

- "Guided meditations for mindful living" by Dr. Alexandra Milspaw
- "Guided meditations for 4-D Healing" by Dr. Alexandra Milspaw
- Jeffrey Thompson psychosensory series – www.scientificsounds.com – bilateral stimulation music to help balance brain activity
- "Sexual Healing" audiobook by Peter Levine, reviews the biology of trauma and how it affects our ability to be present and experience pleasure
- "Retrain Your Pelvic Pain" and "Reigniting Intimacy" workshop series by Dr. Alexandra Milspaw – reviews neurobiology of pain and trauma, how to heal the brain and return to a life of pleasure, intimacy, and fun!

Recommended Apps

- Curable
- Tapping Solution
- Insight Timer
- Headspace
- Paired

Recommended Viewing

- "Proven" documentary series
- "Wisdom of Trauma" by Gabor Mate documentary and interview series

* For more resources, visit my website at www.dralexmilspaw.com.

- "The Tapping Solution" documentary
- Amy Stein's "Healing Pelvic and Abdominal Pain" DVD
- "Anatomy of Trust" by Brene Brown
- "Headspace: A Guide to Meditation" series on Netflix
- TedTalks by Emily Nagoski
- TedTalks by Esther Perel
- "A Very Happy Brain" and "Meditation 2.0" by Dr. Sood on YouTube

Meditative Viewing

- "Moving Art" on Neflix shows a collection of brilliant natural scenes, very colorful and good for the brain.
- "Rivers and tides" with Andy Goldsworthy. He's an artist who creates art with nature and shares his philosophy of life. Simply watching the documentary feels very meditative and soothing.
- "Zenimation" on Disney+. Even if you don't have children you'll enjoy this! Instead of "imagination" it's called "Zennimation" and it's just fabulous. It combines scenes from all these different Disney movies based on themes, such as water scenes, or weather sounds, or landscapes. It's very meditative to watch. I love it.
- "Planet Earth" series with David Attenborough.

Recommended Reading

- *The Hidden Power of Emotional Intuition* by Maya Mendoza
- *Think Again* by Adam Grant
- *The End of Mental Illness* by Daniel Amen
- *Bliss Brain & Mind to Matter* by Dawson Church
- *Better Sex Through Mindfulness* by Lori Brotto
- *Breaking the Habit of Being Yourself* by Joe Dispenza
- *Solving the Autoimmune Puzzle* by Keesha Ewers, MD

- *Getting the Love You Want Workbook* by Hendrix and Hunt
- *Come as You* Are by Emily Nagoski
- *Explain Pain* by Lorimer Moseley
- *Painful Yarns* by Lorimer Moseley
- *Unlearn Your Pain* by Howard Schubiner
- *The Mindful Way Workbook* by Segal et al
- *28 Days to Ecstasy* by Copeland and Link
- *Mindful Relationship Habits* by S.J. Scott and Barrie Davenport
- *Aware* by Daniel Siegel
- *Tapping for Pain Relief* by Nick Ortner
- *Energy Medicine for Women* by Donna Eden
- Mary Ruth Velicki's *Healing Book* series
- *Mindfulness-Based Cognitive Therapy for Depression* by Segal et al
- *Love Sense* by Sue Johnson
- *The Divided Mind* by John Sarno
- *Fear Cure* by Lissa Rankin
- *Healing Painful Sex* by Deborah Coady and Nancy Fish
- *The Heart and Soul of Sex* by Gina Ogden
- *Iyengar Yoga for Motherhood* by Geeta Iyengar, et al
- *Spirit-Centered Relationships* by Gay and Kathleen Hendricks
- *ABC's of Love and Sex* by Gina Ogden
- *Sex, God, and the Conservative Church* by Tina Sellers
- *The Vagina Monologues* by Eve Ensler
- *Insecure at Last* by Eve Ensler
- *Light Therapy* by Martel
- *Brainscapes* by Rebecca Schwarzlose
- *Power and Care* by Tonia Singer and Mattheiu Ricard, editors

- *The Power of Now* by Eckhart Tolle
- *My Grandmother's Hands* by Resmaa Menakem
- *Ancient Sounds for a New Age* by Diane Mandle – book and DVD

Energy Psychology Research and Resources

- www.energypsych.org/page/research_landing
- www.tappingsolution.com
- www.tapwithbrad.com

Sexual Health and Pelvic Pain Informational Websites and Organizations

- pelvicpain.org – International Pelvic Pain Society
- pelvicgym.com
- pelvicguru.com
- paindownthere.com – Educational DVD for pelvic and sexual pain
- aasect.org – American Association of Sexuality Educators, Counselors, and Therapists
- joyofmakinglove.com – Great resource for books, articles, and research on sexual health and wellness
- The Society for the Scientific Study of Sexuality, Inc.
- OMGYES – omgyes.com is a movement to research and provide evidence-based information about the specific ways people increase sexual pleasure
- ichelp.org – Interstitial Cystitis Association
- pudendalhope.org – Pudendal Neuralgia information and resources
- nva.org – National Vulvodynia Association
- www.noigroup.com.au – Neuro-Orthopeadic Institute of Australia – one of the world's leaders in understanding the neurobiology of pain and trauma; check out their books Explain Pain and Painful Yarns

- OBGYN.net's Pelvic Pain page: http://www.obgyn.net/pelvic-pain/
- P.U.R.E. H.O.P.E. — Pelvic and Urological Resources and Education: http://www.pure-hope.org/
- The Woman's Sexual Health Foundation: http://www.twshf.org/
- The Sexual Health Network: http://www.drmitchelltepper.com/sexual_health_network.com/
- Information on Female Sexual Dysfunction: http://www.fsdinfo.org/
- National Institutes of Health – National Library of Medicine: www.nlm.nih.gov/medlineplus/femalesexualdysfunction.html
- Institute for Sexual Medicine – Boston University School of Medicine:www.bumc.bu.edu/sexualmedicine
- Feminist.com: Health and Sexuality links

General Pain Sites

- Neuro-Orthopedic Institute of Australia
- Pain Clinician.com
- Understanding Chronic Pain in 5 Minutes: http://www.pain-ed.com/blog/2013/04/18/a-5-minute-guide-to-understanding-chronic-pain-and-what-you-can-do-about-it/
- American Pain Foundation: http://www.painfoundation.org/
- American Pain Society: http://www.ampainsoc.org/
- The Wasser Pain Management Centre at Mount Sinai Hospital (Toronto):http://www.mtsinai.on.ca/wasser/
- Neuropathic Pain pdf file

Bladder

- Interstitial Cystitis Network: http://www.ic-network.com/
- Interstitial Cystitis Association: http://www.ichelp.org/ – best educational site for average IC sufferer

- International Painful Bladder Association: http://www.painful-bladder.org

Vulvodynia

- Vulvodynia.com: http://www.vulvodynia.com/
- National Vulvodynia Association: http://www.nva.org/
- National Women's Health Resource Center: Vulvodynia article
- Cure Together Open Source Health Resource: Vulvodynia membership page
- Our GYN – For women and their mates, helping each better comprehend gynecological issues: http://www.ourgyn.com/

Recommended Products

- Muse meditation headband and app
- Apollo wrist-band device: apolloneuro.com
- Amy Stein's WellnessX Nature CBD product line
- Ohnut
- Dessert Harvest aloe vera products
- V-Magic Organic healing balm: medicinemamasapothecary.com
- Your Pace Yoga by Dustienne Miller
- Noxicare Natural Pain Relief cream
- SoulSource dilators
- Pure Romance dilators, massage ball, sensate-enhancing gloves, and other gentle products for pleasure
- LifeWave X39 patches: Our bodies create light that can actually stimulate stem cell growth when reflected back to us. LifeWave (lifewave.com) created X39 patches that you can wear on your skin to decrease inflammation and speed up cellular regener

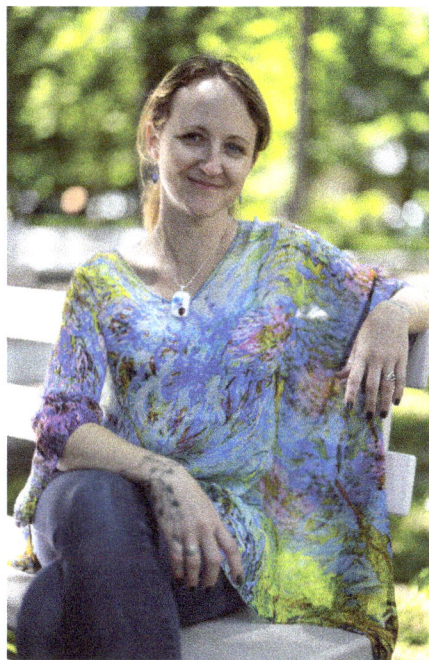

Alexandra T. Milspaw, PhD, MEd, has been practicing counseling and providing educational seminars and trainings since 2007. Dr. Milspaw is a licensed professional counselor in the Commonwealth of Pennsylvania and an AASECT-Certified Sex Therapist. She earned a Master's and Doctoral degree in Human Sexuality from Widener University and a Master's degree in Counseling Psychology and Human Services from Lehigh University. She is certified in Mindfulness-Based Stress Reduction, Neuro-Linguistic Programming, Consulting Hypnosis, and the Explain Pain educational program from the Neuro-Orthopeadic Institute of Australia.

Dr. Milspaw is a Certified 4-D Wheel Practitioner and currently serves as the Vice-President of the 4-D Network (www.4-dnetwork.com). The 4-D Wheel is a four-dimensional approach to understanding, exploring, and discovering all aspects of our human experience. The 4-D Wheel is specifically helpful when addressing not only the effect of chronic pain and trauma on our lives, but also highlights the need for a comprehensive, interdisciplinary treatment approach.

Dr. Milspaw currently serves as the Director of Behavioral Health Services for Pelvic Rehabilitation Medicine – a national, intradisciplinary physiatry clinic specializing in chronic pelvic pain. She also serves as a Board Member and the Chair of the Clinical Foundations Training Course for the International Pelvic Pain Society. She is a co-manager of the Pelvic Messenger Podcast, which provides evidence-based interviews with specialists around the world on chronic pelvic and sexual pain disorders. She also provides annual courses for the Pennsylvania

Bar Institute and Pennsylvania County Bar Associations on the neurobiology of trauma and stress, how to foster resilience and reduce burnout, and how to support trauma victims in the courtroom.

Dr. Milspaw is passionate about bridging the gap between the psychological and medical worlds. She seeks to utilize evidence-based research to highlight the connection between the mental, emotional, physical, and spiritual experiences as a way of empowering clinicians and clients alike to trust the healing potential within everyone. She enjoys reading research about the brain, practicing Iyengar yoga and mindfulness, and playing outside with her two dogs, child, and loving life partner.

"Occasionally a book comes out that opens up subjects that need to be studied. This new book by Dr. Milspaw, *Hello, Down There*, is one of those refreshing books that brings this one taboo subject to the forefront, which helps people to move forward from these once debilitating issues. It is rare to find a book that doesn't just point out the problem but also offers cutting edge techniques and methodologies to help people suffering from chronic pain in the pelvic region. This book gives proven research-based techniques that can help people take control and live the life that they deserve to live. This book by Dr. Milspaw is one of those rare finds for both the practitioner and the user. If you your clients or someone you know suffers from chronic pelvic and sexual pain this book is long overdue and highly recommended. Thank you for bringing this book out at a needed time." —*William D. Horton, Psy. D, MCAP, Founder of National Federation of NeuroLinguistic, https://nfnlp.com*

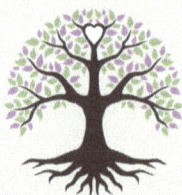

Coming in 2023:

HELLO, UP THERE:
Trauma, disassociation, and the
integration of our parts

www.ingramcontent.com/pod-product-compliance
Lightning Source LLC
Chambersburg PA
CBHW052015030426
42335CB00026B/3153